The
Advanced Practice Nurse
Issues for the New Millennium

Joellen W. Hawkins, RNC, Ph.D., FAAN
Professor, Boston College
Janice A. Thibodeau, RN,C, Ed.D., FAAN
Professor Emerita, University of Connecticut

Fifth Edition

The Tiresias Press, Inc., New York

DEDICATION

In memory of

Sheila A. Packard (1949-1995)

and

Patricia A. Geary (1946-1998)

Advanced practitioners, scholars, and friends

International Standard
Book Number: 0-913292-52-4

Printed in U.S.A.

Preface

THIS BOOK is intended to be both a text for students enrolled in programs preparing them to be advanced practice nurses (APNs) and as a reference for nurses who are already APNs. It translates broad, theoretical concepts into the practical, everyday concerns of nurses in advanced practice roles, and, by analyzing selected issues affecting role implementation, it directs students and nurses already active as advanced practice nurses to assume, examine, and reality test the various aspects of these roles.

The issues addressed here are those concerned with aspects of being an advanced practice nurse beyond the care of patients: negotiating for a job; credentialing for advanced practice; economics of health care delivery, including managed care; legal and regulatory aspects of practice; scope of practice; use of a nursing model for practice; use of change theory; concepts of power, authority, leadership, and sex-role stereotyping; research in advanced practice roles; quality improvement for practice; communication and assertiveness; mentoring; and community assessment for improved or expanded delivery of care by advanced practice nurses.

Acknowledgments

To our students over many years, whose feedback has been invaluable in the development of material for this book, we owe many thanks. Our colleagues in practice have added their support and input as this book evolved.

We are especially grateful to Catherine Collins and Amy Hochler for allowing us to use the evaluation tools they developed for their practice, and to Lynda Clancy and Ellen Robinson for a sample resume and curriculum vitae, respectively.

Most of all, we owe our deepest gratitude to our friends and families for their support of us and tolerance of our seemingly endless projects.

Joellen W. Hawkins

Janice A. Thibodeau

ABOUT THE AUTHORS

Joellen W. Hawkins is a professor at Boston College and a certified obstetrical/gynecological women's health nurse practitioner. Her many books include *Nursing and the American Health Care Delivery System,* The *Dictionary of American Nursing Biography, Protocols for Nurse Practitioners in Gynecologic Settings,* and *Nurse-Social Worker Collaboration in Managed Care: A Model of Community Case Management.*

Janice A. Thibodeau is a professor emerita at the University of Connecticut and a certified adult nurse practitioner. She is the author of *Nursing Models: Analysis and Evaluation.*

Contents

1

Advanced Practice Roles in Nursing

Introduction

The advanced practice role for nurses is not new. The first nurses practicing what is now considered advanced practice nursing were nursing sisters administering anesthesia in 1877 at St. Vincent's Hospital in Erie, Pennsylvania (1, 2). Less than a decade later, nurses in the community were pioneering advanced nursing in public health. The term "public health nurse" was first used by Lillian Wald in 1893 to describe the kind of work her Henry Street Settlement House nurses did when they visited the poor and sick in their homes. Practicing much more independently than hospital nurses, public health nurses at Henry Street and across the United States taught health promotion and disease prevention to school children, workers, citizens in many different community settings, mothers and children through prenatal and well baby clinics, and tenement dwellers served by settlement houses (3). "American nurses saw health visiting as an opportunity for professional independence, status, and economic security. . ." (3, p. 1781). Nurse-midwives were the next group of advanced practice nurses in the U.S.

Thus, advanced practice nursing was not unique to the latter half of the twentieth century when educational preparation moved from service agencies to the academy, although in the years since 1877 it has acquired titles and more formal definitions.

Historical Evolution of Preparation for Advanced Practice and Specialization

Public health nurses led the way in preparing for advanced practice by creating postgraduate courses. In 1906, Charlotte Macleod planned and organized the Training School for Nurses of the Boston

Instructive District Nursing Association (IDNA), the first such course in the country (105). Although the term "advanced practice" would not be used for many years, graduates of postgraduate courses such as those organized by the IDNA prepared nurses for specialist practice and for roles similar to those of today's advanced practice nurses.

By 1931, 137 hospitals were offering postgraduate courses in a wide variety of specialties. Between 1909 and 1912, the first formal postgraduate courses for nurse anesthetists were begun. Nurse-midwives such as Mary Breckinridge were trained in England and other European countries until the Maternity Center Association opened the first U.S. school for them with its affiliate, the Lobenstein Clinic, in New York City (106).

Beginning with postgraduate courses, nurse anesthetists and nurse-midwives went on to develop formal certificate programs for registered nurses based in health care agencies, and in colleges and universities both certificate and degree granting programs were formed. In 1995 there were 95 programs for nurse anesthetists, two-thirds of these in colleges or schools of nursing. Most certificate programs were phased out to meet a 1998 goal that all their accredited programs confer a master's degree. Forty basic and two precertification programs exist for the preparation of nurse-midwives; some are degree granting and others are certificate programs (1, 2, 106).

Nurse Practitioner Education
The first nurse practitioner demonstration project, in 1965, was planned to "determine the safety, efficacy, and quality of a new mode of nursing practice designed to improve health care to children and families and to develop a new nursing role—that of the pediatric nurse practitioner" (4). Loretta Ford was codirector of the project, which took place at the University of Colorado, and she is credited with first using the term nurse practitioner.

By 1998, there were 312 master's programs offering one or more advanced practice options and fewer than a dozen certificate programs (18, 19). A 1998 core curricula survey showed that of the master's programs, 122 offered preparation in one or more nurse practitioner specialty areas (20). Some of these were combined nurse practitioner/clinical nurse specialist programs.

Advanced practice roles in nursing were given a boost by the Nurse Training Act of 1964 (PL 88-581), Title II of the 1968 Health Manpower Act (PL 92-158), and the Nurse Training Act of 1975 (PL 94-63). All of these provided monies for advanced nurse training and the establishment of practitioner programs (9).

In 1971, the Committee of the Secretary of the U.S. Department of Health, Education, and Welfare presented its findings from a study of extended roles for nurses. The report concluded that nurses could assume responsibility for extended roles in primary, acute, and in long-term care; in some cases with additional preparation.

Also in 1971, the University of Washington began a program to prepare family nurse practitioners. Following that example, which became known as PRIMEX, programs were initiated at Cornell-New York Hospital and the University of North Carolina at Chapel Hill (10). Other early programs included the family nurse practitioner program at the University of California, Davis; Boston College's programs in ambulatory care for women and children which were piloted in 1967 and funded by the Josiah Macy Jr. Foundation in 1968; and a program at Wayne State for health nurse clinicians (11).

Recognizing the need for a statement from the professional nursing organization on nursing's expanded role, in 1974 the American Nurses Association (ANA) Congress of Nursing Practice published definitions of the advanced practice roles. These definitions not only addressed matters of the scope of practice but, in addition, stated that skills were to be acquired in continuing education programs following ANA guidelines or in baccalaureate nursing programs (12).

In 1979, the National League for Nursing published a position paper on the education of nurse practitioners, stating that "the nurse practitioner should hold a master's degree in nursing in order to ensure competence and quality care." The statement then emphasized the need for nurses to be educated as practitioners within the formal structure of graduate nursing programs (21) (yet more than two decades later, nurse practitioners do not need to hold a baccalaureate degree to practice in many states) (22). As of 1993, preparation at the graduate level is required to sit for certification examinations offered by the American Nurses Credentialing Center as an adult, family, pediatric, school, or gerontologic nurse practitioner, and by 1998 all generalist certification examinations required a minimum of a baccalaureate degree (23).

Nurse Clinician and Clinical Nurse Specialist Education
In a 1943 speech, Frances Reiter first used the term "nurse clinician," and in 1944, Adelaide A. Mayo defined "clinical nursing specialist" in an article in the *American Journal of Nursing* (5). Dorothy Johnson offered clinical nurse specialists as a solution to the problem of the well-prepared nurse moving away from direct patient care (6). An early master's program to prepare advanced practitioners was developed by Hildegard Peplau at Rutgers University in 1954. It focused on psychiatric nursing (7). Two years later, participants at an interdisciplinary conference agreed that clinical specialists in psychiatric nursing should be prepared at the master's level (8).

Educational preparation for clinical nurse specialists/nurse clinicians evolved in a somewhat different model from that for nurse practitioners. Unlike the deluge of programs to prepare nurse practitioners, no comparable explosion of certificate programs occurred to prepare clinical nurse specialists. Instead, beginning in 1954, master's programs were developed whose focus was advanced clinical practice (7). Most, if not all, of the programs were at the master's level. By 1993, there were 250 master's programs offering preparation in one or more specialty areas for clinical nurse specialists and/or other advanced practice roles.

Among the 312 university and college graduate programs in nursing in 1999, the number offering options to prepare clinical nurse specialists changes almost daily as programs struggle to prepare advanced practice nurses for the twenty-first century (18)

National Credentialing for Advanced Practice

In the late 1960s, certification for advanced practice and certification examinations were developed by the ANA Divisions of Practice. Among the first nurses certified who held advanced practice degrees were those in psychiatric mental health practice (13). Then, in 1976, an ANA program was implemented to provide for certification of nurses as nurse practitioners (14).

Certification for other advanced practice roles followed similar paths. The American Association of Nurse Anesthetists, founded in 1931, began its national certification program around 1941, and the American College of Nurse-Midwives, founded as the American Association of Nurse-Midwives in 1929, established its national certification program in 1971 (1, 2, 106). Thus, in a little over two decades from the first formal nurse practitioner and clinical nurse specialist programs, the concept of role expansion for nurses took hold and gave birth to new definitions of practice and the process of national credentialing for advanced practice.

Preparation for Advanced Practice: Confusion in the Public's Eye

Advanced practice nurses are of four types: nurse anesthetists, nurse-midwives, nurse practitioners, and clinical nurse specialists. There are different educational programs for each of these, with the exception of the blended CNS/NP programs. There is one professional body certifying nurse anesthetists, one for nurse midwives, and several for nurse practitioners and clinical nurse specialists.

Adding to the confusion is the lack of unity in requirements for entry into nurse practitioner programs. Many of the certificate programs require only that one be a registered nurse with a current license to practice. Admission requirements range from physician recommendation and a promise to serve as preceptor to meeting criteria for admission to the graduate school of a university. Upon completion, the individual may receive nothing, a certificate, a baccalaureate degree, or a master's degree. Settings for programs have ranged from physician's offices to hospitals, other health care institutions, schools of nursing, universities and colleges, and schools of public health and medicine. The debate continues concerning the setting for and length of advanced practice programs. Federal guidelines mandate that programs be one year in length in order to qualify for funding. Guidelines for programs have been prepared by the American Nurses Association, the Association of Women's Health, Obstetric, and Neonatal Nurses, the American College of Nurse-Midwives, the American Association of Nurse Anesthetists, and the National Association of Pediatric Nurse Associates and Practitioners. In addition, about two dozen specialty organizations offer certification for specialty and/or advanced practice roles and have promulgated educational standards. Graduates of programs adhering to the guidelines are eligible for certification examinations sponsored by these organizations or their certifying bodies. (See Appendix B.)

Advanced Practice Roles: Blending and Merging
By the mid-1980s, the differences between nurse practitioners and clinical nurse specialists were blurring. Certificate practitioner programs were declining and the number of master's programs was rising.

The results of the clinical nurse specialist and nurse practitioner core curricula survey of 1990 demonstrated that, at the master's level, preparation for both roles is quite similar. Differences exist in clinical content (pharmacology, primary care, history taking and physical assessment, nutrition, and health promotion in nurse practitioner programs) and in clinical settings (with more secondary and tertiary for clinical specialists) (24).

In a working document for the Council of Clinical Nurse Specialists and the Council of Primary Care Nurse Practitioners of the American Nurses Association, Sparacino and Durand laid out the similarities and differences in the two advanced practice roles (27). In 1990, the two councils merged, reflecting a transition to designation as nurses in advanced practice (28). Of course, such a merger did not occur without dissent, and since that time several new nurse practitioner organizations have been formed, as has the National Association of Clinical Nurse Specialists (17).

Some have argued that clinical specialists should move toward the nurse practitioner name and role, in part because of the power base and public recognition associated with the title nurse practitioner (30). In several studies, merging of roles is evident. Elder and Bullough (31) surveyed graduates of nurse practitioner and clinical nurse specialist programs and found fewer differences than the literature might suggest and a general consensus that the roles should merge. The core curriculum study of 1990 supported congruence in master's preparation between the two roles, as noted earlier (24). Diers argued that we no longer have "generalized practice," and that advanced nurse practitioners should be prepared for specialty practice at the master's level (32). The greatest differentiation between clinical nurse specialists and nurse practitioners occurred earlier when education programs developed on divergent paths: certificate and master's. With convergence of those paths, merging of the roles becomes clearer.

Several other changes have propelled us toward merging these two advanced practice roles. Unlike the roles of nurse-midwives and nurse anesthetists, nurse practitioner and clinical nurse specialist roles are far less delineated. The differences between these roles blur as settings for practice become less important as providers move across boundaries, managed care systems grow, lengths of stay in acute care settings shorten, and more care moves back into the community. "The way we define specialties and roles may be becoming obsolete" (25). A merged role could maximize the expertise brought to the advanced practice role and make the role more viable (26, 33).

Tilting for Advanced Practice
In professional nursing literature, as in that of other professions, the

lay press, and in legislation, consensus grew in the 1990s that nurses in advanced practice—nurse practitioners, clinical nurse specialists, certified nurse-midwives, and certified registered nurse anesthetists—should be collectively referred to as advanced practice nurses (15, 22, 85, 102). "Advanced practice nurse (APN)" is "an umbrella term given to a registered nurse who has met advanced educational and practice requirements, usually at the master's level, beyond the basic nursing education and licensing required of all RNs" (109). The American Nurses Association and the American Association of Critical Care Nurses have adopted the term advanced practice nurse (111). The American Association of Colleges of Nursing in 1994 endorsed advanced practice nurse as "an umbrella term appropriate for a licensed registered nurse prepared at the graduate degree level as either a clinical specialist, nurse anesthetist, nurse-midwife, or nurse practitioner" (108, p. 1). The National League for Nursing has recommended merging two advanced practice roles—clinical nurse specialist and nurse practitioner—under a single title, and the Division of Nursing of the U.S. Public Health Service, Department of Health and Human Services, has agreed that by 2010 the roles will be merged (103). Many states are using the term advanced practice nurse in new or proposed legislation authorizing advanced practice under nurse practice acts and in propagating regulations for prescription writing and third-party reimbursement (22, 29).

Debates over titles are considered by some to be counterproductive (107). Others predict that in the new millennium only "the most flexible will be here to practice nursing" (110). Starck pointed out that nurses seem obsessed with titles: "What other profession redefines what it calls itself as often as we do?" (104)

Practice Settings

When Lucille Kinlein became an independent practitioner around three decades ago, she was declaring to the public that she, as a nurse, had something unique and special to offer to patients (34). Numerous other nurses have followed her example and have met with varied success (35, 36). Independent practice is only one option for advanced practice nurses, however. Settings for practice and practice arrangements vary widely among those nurses calling themselves and practicing as nurse practitioners, clinical nurse specialists, nurse-midwives, and nurse anesthetists.

Figures on the numbers of advanced practice nurses are difficult to obtain. In a Division of Nursing study, investigators used position titles, national certification data, and formal preparation for the role to obtain their statistics (37). By 1998, 48,237 nurse practitioners and 41,893 clinical nurse specialists were estimated to be employed in the U.S. Through membership data, the American College of Nurse-Midwives put their numbers at 7,000 in 1999, and the American Association of Nurse Anesthetists places their numbers at over 27,000 (2).

Practice settings for these advanced practice nurses include hospitals (federal, psychiatric, long- and short-term general and all care settings within those hospitals), nursing homes, schools of nursing, public health agencies, college and university student health services, public and private schools, early intervention programs, senior centers, work sites, prisons, ambulatory care agencies, including those under managed care arrangements, self-employment (including nurse managed centers), and in patients' homes. Clinical nurse specialists are employed in the same settings, but in differing proportions, particularly those holding positions in hospitals (29). Nurse anesthetists administer over 65% of anesthetics in the United States, are the sole providers of anesthesia in 75% of rural hospitals, and work in all health care settings where anesthesia is given (81). Nurse-midwives are most likely to practice in hospital clinics, private offices, and public clinics; they also practice in HMOs and birth centers (40, 79). With managed care systems controlling an increasing proportion of the health care market, more advanced practice nurses are employed by or contract with these systems. Psychiatric nurses with a master's degree or above, in many cases indicating clinical specialization in psychiatric-mental health nursing, are employed in outpatient facilities, state and county hospitals, private psychiatric hospitals, residential treatment centers for emotionally disturbed children, other types of residential facilities, VA psychiatric organizations, mental health care organizations, home care, and multiservice mental health organizations (15, 37, 80, 95, 106). The 1990s added other settings for nurses with advanced practice preparation: shelters for the homeless and for battered women, soup kitchens, and health care programs for homeless persons (38).

A number of authors have suggested that advanced practice nurses must learn to market themselves to potential patients including managed care systems. Some of their articles focus on the role of advanced practitioners in private practice, others on new or enlarging patient groups such as older adults, or on nontraditional settings such as ambulatory centers managed by other than physicians (39, 42).

Towers (43) reported from a national survey of nurse practitioners that fewer than half of the respondents market themselves. When they do, they use pamphlets, the yellow pages, newspaper ads, and special referral arrangements. Hershey (44) might have expanded his statement to include all advanced practice nurses when he wrote that "an aggressive attitude aimed at capturing for nursing anything that physicians might be willing to yield sole dominion over enhances nursing as a profession and the economic opportunity for nurse practitioners."

In chapters to follow, we discuss marketing ourselves as advanced practice nurses, including preparing a resume or curriculum vitae, creating a professional portfolio, and managing an interview.

Primary Activities of Nurses in Advanced Practice

For *nurse practitioners,* primary activities include screening, physical and psychosocial assessment, follow-up when deviations from normal are detected, continuity of care, health promotion, problem-centered services related to diagnosis, identification, and mobilization of resources, health education, and patient and group advocacy.

Nurse practitioners may be involved with aspects of primary, secondary, and tertiary care (45, 46, 48, 114). Functions identified in the longitudinal study of nurse practitioners include taking a health history, performing a physical examination, patient care management, surveillance of well persons, and illness care (49). In a national survey of 5,964 nurse practitioners, Towers (50) reported that nurse practitioners "manage pharmacologic therapeutics in all fifty states, across all specialties, and in all locales..." Practice patterns of nurse practitioners have been studied and add to our knowledge of roles (83).

Case management can be a role suitable for all advanced practice nurses. Components of the role include selecting patients, planning care for cost effectiveness and for optimal outcomes, procuring and coordinating care, collaborating with other members of the health care team, and monitoring and evaluating outcomes, in addition to performing physical assessments, selecting laboratory and other diagnostic tests, and prescribing medications (45). Nurse practitioners also engage in many of the indirect roles of clinical nurse specialists.

The *clinical nurse specialist's* role encompasses a number of direct and indirect care aspects. In one review of role expectations, the authors found the clinician or direct care role to be foremost (51), with indirect roles including consultant-liaison, staff advocate, peer educator, change agent, policy analyst, patient educator, product evaluator, researcher, supervisor, and mentor and corporate/ community advanced practice nurse (29, 47, 52, 53, 54, 55, 56, 57, 84, 95). Another analysis of the role activities corroborates these findings and adds the category of professional development which includes self-directed learning activities, continuing education, and writing for publications other than those associated with research (58).

Nurse-midwives provide prenatal, intrapartal, and postpartum care, and well woman care including family planning. They may also have administrative, education, case manager and/or consultation roles. Suturing, prescribing, and preventive care such as immunizations are common activities. On call time is required of many nurse-midwives for deliveries and for triaging pregnant and postpartum patients (63, 106).

Nurse anesthetists evaluate patients for anesthetic agents and monitor patients' responses to anesthetics administered by themselves or other professionals. They evaluate postanesthesia recovery and facilitate diagnostic, therapeutic, emergency, and surgical interventions. They are also educators, administrators, consultants, and case managers, particularly for patients with acute or chronic pain or chronic ventilatory problems. (2, 48).

All of these functions relate to the scope of practice statements that have been generated by various professional organizations in attempts to provide guidelines on what it is that nurses in advanced practice roles do for and with their patients that is unique and different. (See Appendix A.)

Scope of Practice
Scope of practice statements are based on what is legally allowable in each state under its nurse practice act. They do, however, go beyond the law in some states, as they are prepared by national professional organizations. Their intention is to provide guidelines for the practice of nursing under special conditions and with advanced preparation. These statements also may be interpreted as indicators of the expectations employers and patients may have of those who call themselves nurse practitioners, nurse-midwives, clinical nurse specialists, or nurse anesthetists, indicating a particular target population. In reviewing scope of practice statements, however, it is important to recognize that they are guidelines rather than mandates. Fagin (59) has written, ". . . nursing's scope of practice must be viewed as fluid and evolutionary." In a study of specialization in nursing, Styles points out the value to the profession of empowerment through expertise (61). Advanced practice nurses can capitalize on the expertise they possess. But we need to document and communicate that expertise.

In the 1970s, as the advanced practice movement gained momentum and programs proliferated, a number of the professional organizations, both nursing and medical, set about the task of developing scope of practice statements and guidelines for educational preparation.

The American Nurses Association took the lead in developing program guidelines and scope of practice statements for college health, geriatric, adult and family, and pediatric nurse practitioners. A list of such publications is included in Appendix A. Each of these guidelines and statements addresses practice activities and settings.

Concurrently, scope of practice statements were developed for specialty advanced practice. The documents may also include statements about professional responsibility, interprofessional relationships, and patient advocacy. Various divisions on practice, later renamed the councils of the ANA but now defunct, prepared the early versions of the scope documents. The one on college health is co-authored by the American College Health Association. The guidelines for educational programs address issues such as goals, planning, services and facilities, faculty, course content, admission of students, length, and evaluation. ANA continues to promulgate scope of practice statements for advanced practice nurses, sometimes in collaboration with other specialty nursing organizations.

The National Association of Pediatric Nurse Associates and Practitioners (NAPNAP) and the American Academy of Pediatrics in 1975 issued a joint statement on the scope of practice, functions, and responsibilities of pediatric nurse associates and practitioners. In 1974, the ANA issued a scope of practice statement for pediatric nurse practitioners, updating it in 1996. NAPNAP continues to update the scope of practice statement for pediatric nurse practitioners.

The Nurses' Association of the American College of Obstetricians and Gynecologists, or NAACOG (as of 1993 its name became the Association of Women's Health, Obstetric, and Neonatal Nurses; its acronym: AWHONN), has taken an active role in defining practice for women's health and maternal and newborn care. In 1979, in collaboration with the American Academy of Family Physicians, the American Academy of Pediatrics, the American College of Obstetricians and Gynecologists, and NAPNAP, NAACOG issued a statement on the role definition, description, and educational guidelines for obstetric-gynecologic women's health nurse practitioners, updating the document in 1984, 1990, and 1996, the latter in collaboration with the National Association of Nurse Practitioners in Reproductive Health (NANPRH, now NPWH).

NAACOG also issued statements on the expanded role of health professionals in obstetric and gynecologic care (1980), definitions of nursing titles (including nurse practitioners), and a definition of primary health care (1979). AWHONN has issued statements on scope of practice and educational preparation of neonatal nurse practitioners (1997) in collaboration with the National Association of Neonatal Nurses (NANN) and nurses specializing in infertility.

The American College of Nurse-Midwives administers national certification examinations, issues scope of practice statements for nurse-midwifery practice, and sets standards for educational programs, which exist both as certificate granting entities and as part of master's degree preparation.

The practice of nurse anesthetists is regulated by state statutes, policies of institutions, and scope of practice and certification requirements of the American Association of Nurse Anesthetists. Educational guidelines are propagated by the Council on Accreditation of Nurse Anesthesia Educational Programs. (2)

Many of the more than 30 organizations that certify nurses also have prepared scope of practice statements in addition to those cited here. Notable among these is the American Association of Critical Care Nurses which, in concert with the ANA, issued standards of practice and scope of practice statements for acute care nurse practitioners in 1995. Some, of course, do not specify advanced practice with educational preparation in a certificate or graduate program (60).

In 1995, the ANA issued the revised version of Nursing's Social Policy Statement. According to this statement, "Nursing's scope of practice is dynamic and evolves with changes in the phenomena of concern, in knowledge about various interventions' effects on patient or group outcomes, or in the political environment, legal conditions, and cultural and demographic patterns in society." This policy statement addressed the issue of specialists within nursing and/or recognized those nurses prepared at the graduate level and/or those certified by ANA.

The nurse preparing for or practicing in an advanced practice role must be familiar with those scope of practice documents pertinent to her/his area of expertise. In addition to the state nurse practice acts, scope of practice statements delineate expectations, roles, and responsibilities which may reasonably be part of the practice of such a practitioner. They may provide the basis for preparing a job description, for materials to educate the public about what an advanced practice nurse does, and as the basis for evaluation of practice.

It is interesting to note the intrusion of physicians and physician organizations into the arena and their attempts to define and delineate what nurses may do. The American Academy of Pediatrics, the American College of Obstetricians and Gynecologists, and other physician groups have issued several policy statements on the practice of nurses. These include a policy on the pediatric nurse associate, a definition of pediatric nurse practitioners/associates, and a statement on the use of school nurse practitioners.

We as nurses must be assertive in controlling our practice and defining what constitutes nursing. If we abdicate these responsibilities, others will take over. The efforts of the American Nurses Association and its constituent members are important to the nursing profession as a whole. Supporting the ANA, state nurses associations, and/or other specialty groups for advanced practice is one way to assure that nurses retain control over nursing.

Interdisciplinary Aspects of the Role
Since the formal conceptualization of the advanced practice roles in 1954 and 1965, collaboration has been an integral part of those

roles. It is inherent in the definition of primary care. According to the definition prepared by the ANA Congress for Nursing Practice, one component of the role is "interprofessional consultation" (62). In many states, advanced practice nurses (some or all) must work with a collaborating physician (22). Mauksch has stated that the nurse/physician dyad is most important to patient care. Whereas she viewed physicians as focusing on illness, diagnosis, treatment, and curing, nurses focus on wellness, assessment and interventions, caring, comforting, teaching, counseling, and coordinating. She went on to state that physicians must move toward viewing nurses as colleagues, to saying "we" rather than "I," from "what's in it for me" to "what is best for the client," and to learn respect for patients as human beings (64). Mauksch pointed out that physicians are not always interested in collaboration, however, and may even actively oppose nurse practitioners (65).

One of the reasons that interdisciplinary collaboration is so important to the roles in advanced practice is the responsibility for continuity and coordination of care inherent in providing primary care or in case management. It becomes a critical issue for nurses serving as primary care providers or case managers because overlap of functions is more obvious in these roles than for nurses in other areas. Additionally, nurses now are prepared to assume responsibility for components of care that were previously the sole domain of physicians, such as physical examinations. Conflicts over territoriality are common as health care providers are reluctant to yield turf or recognize the expertise of others (66). As Challela (67) noted, nurses have often relied on being liked rather than on being evaluated objectively for the contributions they make to patient care based on expertise and knowledge.

The now defunct National Joint Practice Commission (1972-1981) defined joint practice as "nurses and physicians collaborating as colleagues to provide patient care" (69). To adopt the view that nurses, physicians, or any one type of professional health care provider can provide for all of the health care needs of an individual, family, group, or community over an extended period of time is exceedingly myopic. Thus, nurses in advanced practice roles have been forced, by the very nature of their practice as case managers, to seek collaborative working relationships with other providers, particularly physicians.

When the National Joint Practice Commission began to study joint practice in 1973, efforts were made to identify such practices in order to collect data. Over 250 nurse/physician practices were identified (74). Selected cases from the study are published in *Together* (74). They illustrate how physicians and nurses can collaborate as colleagues with the common goal of giving sensitive, high quality care for patients in a variety of settings, from suburbia to the mountains of Tennessee, utilizing a number of models for the relationships, ranging from teams to a single nurse/physician duo. Current interest is reflected in literature on collaborative practice (70, 72).

A variety of associations is possible. Nurses may establish joint practices with other providers. They may utilize, and in turn be utilized by, others as consultants. Nurses in advanced practice may be employed by physicians, clinics, health maintenance organizations and other managed care systems, nursing homes, or other institutions not controlled by nurses, or may contract with agencies or institutions to obtain certain services for their patients or to deliver certain services. Advanced practice nurses also employ physicians and/or other health professionals or are in joint practices with profit sharing. It is possible for nurses to form partnerships or corporations to provide a wide range of services including anesthesia, nurse-midwifery care, well woman care, and home care (2, 36, 63). Relationships may also be much less formal, as when all providers are employees of an agency or institution such as a community health center, clinic, or HMO.

Joint practice between nurses and physicians has received much attention in the literature (68). Since "nursing and medicine have the longest traditions and the greatest numbers," it is not surprising that attention is focused on the relationship between these two groups of professionals (71). The nurse practitioner role as it evolved in the 1960s grew out of a collaborative effort between a physician and a nurse faculty person interested in the care of children in the community. Many of the early programs utilized and even required physician preceptors since there were, of course, few nurse preceptors available at first. Because clinical nurse specialists evolved out of advanced practice and specialty roles in secondary and tertiary settings, preceptorships were often less troublesome to find among nurses. An exception might be psychiatric-mental health nursing with blurring of roles as primary therapist with the psychiatrist, psychologist, and psychiatric social worker (8).

It is important to recognize and acknowledge that, in a sense, the roles of physician and nurse *are* competitive. Nurses are and will be competing for office space, organizational support, a share of the health care dollar, designation as primary care providers, contracts with managed care organizations, and a voice in decision making for health policies, including "state licensure laws and federal payment schemes" at all levels (76, p. 25). Nurses and physicians must, however, be collaborative and collegial as well as competitive if goals for patient care are to be met (71).

Collaborative relationships with other members of the health care team are inherent in and essential to the role of nurses in advanced practice. Whether these are intra- or interdisciplinary, such relationships are implied in the delivery of primary care, in at least some examples of secondary and tertiary care, and in case management models. Interpretation of the role of the nurse to other providers is an important component of the collaborative process. Many examples exist in the literature to support collaborative interdisciplinary practice for APNs in a variety of settings (41, 49, 75).

The 1980 ANA publication, *Nursing: A Social Policy Statement* (63), defines collaboration as "true partnership," one in which both sides have and value power, recognize and accept separate and combined spheres of responsibility and activity, mutually safeguard the interests of each, and share common goals. Such a relationship thrives on the richness each lends to the other because of the strengths and uniqueness each can contribute to the whole. One of the goals for advanced practice nurses in role development is establishing such relationships with other health care professionals.

Acceptance of Advanced Practice Nurses by Other Health Care Professionals

Advanced practice nurses experience varying degrees of acceptance of their roles by other providers. In the early years, a number of surveys and studies were conducted of nurse practitioners and clinical nurse specialists which looked at the acceptance of such nurses by others, in particular by physicians. Simmons and Rosenthal (77) found that nurse practitioners whom they interviewed perceived trust on the part of some physicians and total rejection by others. Those who perceived distrust characterized their working relationships with physicians as good, but hastened to add that they work with a biased sample of physicians.

The acceptance of pediatric nurse practitioners by pediatricians was explored in a study conducted by Claiborn and Walton (78). They found that physicians in nonprivate practice and subspecialty practice and those working with poverty-level patients were more accepting, as were those who were younger and had been in practice a short time. The physicians who were rated as antipractitioner felt the concept would alter physician-patient relationships and that quality would be sacrificed for quantity.

Nurse practitioners and their employers agreed that resistance from other health providers constitutes one barrier to role development. Similarly, clinical nurse specialists identified rejection by other providers as an impediment to integration into the system and role implementation in general (82).

One component of a study of clinical nurse specialists in collaborative practice was physician acceptance. The authors of the study found that the physicians were satisfied with collaboration, and the clinical nurse specialists in the sample felt physicians' expectations were appropriate (62).

In an extensive review of barriers to practice for advanced practice nurses, Safriet concluded in 1992 that a chaotic regulatory maze, unique to each state, is a major obstacle. Some responsibility for the chaos must be attributed to physicians who, in Safriet's view, know little more about the abilities of advanced practice nurses than do legislators (15). Other investigators corroborate this lack of information about the roles of advanced practice nurses (73). Over the past few years the regulatory barriers have eroded as many states have revised laws on the practice of advanced practice nurses (22, 76).

The most significant challenges encountered by advanced practice nurses today are "an increase in the competitive chaos of the marketplace." According to Safriet's analysis, advanced practice nurses face obstacles from "private contracting, market share, and capital requirements. . . . [From] closed panels to physician-dominated contracting arrangements with integrated delivery systems, APNs and other nonphysician providers face new nongovernmental market-based impediments to their practice." One survey of nurse practitioners' arrangements with managed care plans exists in the literature (86, 76, p. 25).

Relationships between advanced practice nurses, other providers, and care systems can be characterized in a number of ways. Those APNs who are primarily guests in a physician's private practice or employees in managed care systems will find themselves constrained in role development. Control is not shared but remains primarily with the host and rules are established by the host.

The nurse may serve in a gatekeeper role for an agency, or that position may be relegated to another provider. These settings tend to be highly formalized and have many structural controls built into the system. Often the consistent providers are the nurses whose investment is greater than that of the transients in the system. Role development may then be constrained by the system. On the other hand, if nurses have longevity as providers, they may use the advantage of accrued seniority and familiarity to establish the rules, develop protocols, and control their own practice in a collegial relationship with physicians. Telepractice, too, is changing the rules and regulations for practice by all health professionals who potentially could be practicing across state or even country boundaries (76). The nurse whose role includes management activities may also find that she or he represents stability within the provider population. A survey of clinical nurse specialists three to five years after graduation demonstrated roles in administration, especially in planning and policy making (87). Advantages may result from continuity of contact with patients and investment in the position over time. Role development and acceptance as a colleague by other providers may result from the nurse's position as a manager and the relative power within the system (86).

When interviewing for a job, awareness of the possible patterns of relationships will enable the advanced practice nurse to assess the potential for role development, barriers to role implementation, and acceptance by other providers in a work environment (see Chapter 9). To some degree, patterns can be predicted if one makes inquiries about organization's structure and process, caseload assignment, consultation, economic terms, and the philosophy of care. Exploring the controls which regulate the access of each provider to patients will help the nurse evaluate how the nurse's advanced role will be accepted by those with whom she or he will be working most closely and what potential there will be for change (62, 86).

Socialization into the Role

Assuming roles that are only a few decades old and which are still a source of confusion for both the public and other providers is an awesome prospect. The need for students preparing for advanced practice roles to explore components of the role beyond hands-on patient care is evident in their obsession with questions such as: How do I define my role to others? What do I do if I am expected to perform activities for which I have not been prepared? Identifying generic professional behaviors can be helpful in analyzing advanced practice roles (88).

The National Organization of Nurse Practitioners Faculty (NONPF) has been working in collaboration with the American Association of Colleges of Nursing (AACN) on core competencies for nurse practitioners (112). The National Council of State Boards of Nursing (NCSBN) has developed model family nurse practitioner guidelines (113). These documents are useful for faculty, students, and clinical preceptors.

One of the problems in preparing nurses as advanced practice specialists and socializing them into the role is the paucity of faculty with active practices who can act as role models for collegiality in practice with other providers, especially physicians (89). In 1977, the Robert Wood Johnson Foundation initiated funding for a yearlong fellowship program to prepare faculty in primary care. These fellowships afforded faculty the opportunity to prepare for and practice the role of primary care provider in a collaborative relationship (90). By increasing the emphasis on clinical practice and reward systems for faculty who maintain an active practice, the availability of models can be increased.

Innovative approaches to faculty practice through joint appointments (91), shared practices with other providers, demonstration interdisciplinary teams, and the creation of nursing wellness centers and other nurse-managed practice models (46) all provide means for faculty to carry a practice and retain clinical competence. The availability of faculty role models enhances the educational process and socializes students into all aspects of the role of the advanced practice nurse, clinical and nonclinical.

Students in graduate programs need opportunities to explore the nonclinical aspects of their roles. After the initial focus on patient assessment and management skills, students need to move on to role construction (92). At the same time, it is important to recognize that the nurse in advanced practice must ultimately define his or her role and realize that the role is "a negotiative process undertaken in the context of an actual work situation" (93).

Part of socialization involves the opportunity for role practice and role negotiation. These experiences can be built into an educational program. The art of negotiation is useful at all levels of practice, from one-on-one relationships to the macro system level and can be taught in graduate programs (94) (see Chapter 5). Opportunities to apply one's knowledge in as realistic a setting as possible are critical to learning about one's role (89, 92).

Some of the role-related issues which have been identified during the process of role acquisition include increased responsibility for patient care inherent in providing primary, secondary, or tertiary care or serving as a case manager; changing relationships with other providers, particularly physicians, and with care systems; alterations in relationships with significant others (92); public concepts of what an advanced practice nurse is and does; and how to negotiate the role without detriment to employment opportunities. Discussion about role definition and negotiation should be part of the educational process for becoming an advanced practice nurse (89, 92, 97). Such discussion might also be an integral part of continuing education programs for advanced practice nurses and of professional organizations. Indeed, we should not forget the need that nurses already in advanced practice roles have to prepare for role advancement opportunities (89, 98). Faculty might even facilitate mentor relationships for students (see Chapter 7), as well as nurture the preceptors who are so critical to the education of advanced practice nurses (96).

Advanced Practice Around the Globe

Advanced practice nursing is not unique to the United States. In many countries, nurse-midwifery is an integral part of basic nursing education, as the need for providers is so great. Likewise, nurses may be taught to administer anesthesia so that surgery is available in small and remote hospitals. Advanced practice as it has come to be defined in the United States is evolving around the globe.

During the 1980s, nurse practitioner programs in Canada were canceled, reflecting an oversupply of physicians. In June, 1992, the

Canadian Nurses Association (CNA) issued a paper raising issues about reopening the nurse practitioner programs and defining the scope of practice and educational preparation (115). In 1995, the College of Nurses of Ontario (CNO) set standards of practice for nurse practitioners, criteria for registration in the Extended Class of practice for nurses, and listed universities offering programs for primary care nurse practitioners. The Ministry of Health for the province then promulgated laws and regulations (116, 117, 118). As the role evolves under close scrutiny within and among the provinces, data from one study suggest a complementary role for nurse practitioners in primary care (119).

In Australia, the nurse practitioner role is evolving, raising questions of preparation and issues of autonomy, independent practice, credentialing, and regulation of practice (120). New Zealand has nurse-midwives and no legal or practice restrictions barring independent practice by nurses. To date, there are no independent prescribing privileges for nurses in New Zealand, but nurses can prescribe through a cumbersome collaborative arrangement with physicians. There is, however, no recognition for reimbursement by the major insurance companies. Nonetheless, New Zealand nurse entrepreneurs are pushing independent practice (121).

For nearly two decades, nurse practitioners have been developing an advanced practice role in the United Kingdom, whose citizens have long been familiar with advanced practice nurse in the role of nurse-midwife. The Royal College of Nursing has played a role in formalizing education for nurse practitioners and in defining the scope of practice (122, 127). As in Canada, some proponents envision a complementary role with general practitioners (123), while others suggest the importance of autonomous practice (122, 124).

In late 1997, an international conference on nurse practitioners was held in the Netherlands. An experimental program is underway at the Groningen University Hospital there to implement the nurse practitioner's role. The program has the full support from the country's Minister of Health (125).

Israel is currently struggling with issues of regulation of nursing practice and of differentiation of nurses by practice site (hospital, clinics) and inclusion of nurse-midwives under one licensing scheme or a separate recognition (126). Like many other countries, diffentiation among levels of nursing preparation and practice is a major issue, clouded by functional roles and specialization and often disparate levels of preparation among those who may legally call themselves nurses.

These are but some of the examples of the growth and development of new advanced practice roles around the globe. The issues reflect those we have struggled with and the emerging models have something to offer countries from the embryonic to the mature stages in their development of advanced practice nursing.

Summary

The content and process of role implementation are important issues for the individual practicing in an advanced role. "Nursing is not second-class medicine, but first-class health care" (99). Ford has pointed out that the role of the nurse in advanced practice is not well understood and that nurses themselves are not always clear about their roles and are, therefore, allowing the system to use them inappropriately (100).

Role conflicts and role negotiations are a way of life for these nurses. We can expect to expend considerable energy trying to get physicians, other providers, managed care systems, legislators, and the public to understand who we are and what we have to offer. Those of us who serve as role models, as faculty and preceptors, must help prepare our students for the problems inherent in role change. Support for and interpretation of new roles is, at least in part, the responsibility of nursing leadership. Nurses in advanced practice have a great deal to offer to the public in expertise and wellness and illness care. We are the ones responsible for delineating and defining our roles and scope of practice, for determining settings, and for educating other providers and the general public (48, 101).

In the chapters to follow, we will discuss use of a conceptual model for practice that reflects what is unique in the care we offer as advanced practice nurses (Chapter 2). Putting one's model into practice requires a thorough knowledge of the concepts of power, politics, and leadership, discussed in Chapter 6. Increasingly, the chaos in health care requires that advanced practice nurses be competitive in the health care marketplace. Strategies to help the advanced practice nurse become more assertive are discussed in Chapter 5. Since a conceptual model lends direction to practice, the advanced practitioner must be a change agent who understands the theory and process of change. The boundaries of practice are influenced by the legal and regulatory systems at the state and federal levels. These are discussed in Chapters 4 and 10.

By facilitating the research process, the advanced practitioner is assisted in developing prescriptive theories to guide clinical practice and improve the quality of care. Quality improvement and research are discussed in Chapters 11 and 3. Chapters 7 and 9 focus on the practical aspects of negotiating an employment contract and career development and advancement, with special emphasis on mentorship. Chapter 8 continues the discussion of employment with a focus on the economics of advanced practice. The closing chapter discusses the role of the advanced practice nurse in improving health for all by conducting community assessment.

REFERENCES

1.   Bankert, M. (1989). *Watchful Care: A History of America's Nurse Anesthe-tists.* New York: Continuum.
2.   Waugaman, W.R. & Foster, S.D. (1995). CRNAs: An enviable legacy of patient service. *Advanced Practice Nursing Quarterly 1(1):21-28.*
3.   Buhler-Wilkerson, K. (1993) Bringing care to the people: Lillian Wald's legacy to public health nursing. *American Journal of Public Health 83, 1778-1786.*
4.   Ford, L.C. & Silver, H.K. (1967). Expanded role of the nurse in child care. *Nursing Outlook 15:43-45.*
5.   Mayo, A.A. (1944). Advanced courses in clinical nursing. *American Journal of Nursing 44(6):579-585.*

6. Beecroft, P.C. & Papenhausen, J.L. (1989). Who is a clinical nurse specialist? *Clinical Nurse Specialist 4(3):103-104.*
7. Montemuro, M.A. (1987). The evolution of the clinical nurse specialist: Response to the challenge of professional nursing practice. *Clinical Nurse Specialist 1(3):106-ll0.*
8. Martin, E.J. (1985). "A specialty in decline?" *Journal of Professional Nursing 9(1):48-53.*
9. Levine, E. (1977). What do we know about nurse practitioners? *American Journal of Nursing 77:1799-1803.*
10. Walker, A.E. (1972). PRIMEX—the family nurse practitioner program. *Nursing Outlook 20:28-31.*
11. Preparing nurses for family health care. (1972). *Nursing Outlook 20:53-56.*
12. American Nurses Association Congress for Nursing Practice (1974). Definition: Nurse practitioner, nurse clinician and clinical nurse specialist. Kansas City, MO: American Nurses' Association.
13. Jones, F.M. (1981). ANA's certification for specialization. In: J.C. McCloskey & H.K. Grace (Eds.), *Current Issues in Nursing.* Boston: Blackwell Scientific. pp. 353-359.
14. Allen, E.A. (1977). Credentialing of continuing education nurse practitioner programs. In: A.A. Bliss and E.D. Cohen (Eds.), *The New Health Professionals.* Germantown, MD: Aspen. p. 83.
15. Safriet, B.J. (1992). Health care dollars and regulatory sense. *Yale Journal on Regulation 9:417-488.*
16. Stewart, I.M. (1931). Trends in nursing education. *American Journal of Nursing, 31(5):601-614.*
17. Davidson, S.B. (1998). NACNS news. *Clinical Nurse Specialist 12(4):135-136.*
18. AACN/NONPF survey shows NP production on the rise. (1998, May). *Clinician News, 29.*
19. NP educational programs. (1998). *Clinician Reviews 8(12):92-106.*
20. Forbes, K.E., Rafson, J., Spross, J.A. & Kozlowski, D. (1990). Clinical nurse specialist and nurse practitioner core curricula survey results. *The Nurse Practitioner 15(4):43;46-48.*
21. National League for Nursing position statement on the education of nurse practitioners. (1979). New York: National League for Nursing.
22. Pearson, L.J. (1999). Annual update of how each state stands on legislative issues affecting advanced nursing practice. *Nurse Practitioner 24(1):16-83.*
23. American Nurses Association (1989). Directory of Accredited Organizations and Continuing Education Certificate Programs Preparing Nurse Practitioners. Kansas City, MO; ANA.
24. Forbes, K.E., Rafson, J., Spross, J.A. & Kozlowski, D. (1990). Clinical nurse specialist and nurse practitioner core curricula survey results. *Nurse Practitioner 15(4), 43, 46-48.*
25. Cronenwett, L.R. (1995). Molding the future of advanced practice nursing. *Nursing Outlook 43(3), 113.*
26. Busen, N.H. & Engleman, S.G. (1996). The CNS with practitioner prepara-

tion: An emerging role in advanced practice nursing. *Clinical Nurse Specialist 10(3):145-150.*

27.   Sparacino, P. & Durand, B.A. (1986). Specialization in advanced practice. *CPHCNP Newsletter 9:(2):3-4.*

28.   Hawkins, J.E. & Rafson, J. (1991). ANA council merger creates council of nurses in advanced practice. *Clinical Nurse Specialist 5(3):131-132.*

29.   Wood, C.M., Caldwell, M.A., Cusck, M.K., et al. (1996). Clinical nurse specialists in California: Who claims the title? *Clinical Nurse Specialist 10(6):283-291.*

30.   Hanson, C. & Martin, L.L. (1990). The nurse practitioner and clinical nurse specialist: Should the roles be merged? *Journal of the American Academy of Nurse Practitioners 2(1):2-9.*

31.   Elder, R.G. & Bullough, B. (1990). Nurse practitioners and clinical nurse specialists: Are the role merging? *Clinical Nurse Specialist 4(2):78-84.*

32.   Diers, D. (1985). Preparation of practitioners, clinical specialists, and clinicians. *Journal of Professional Nursing 1(1):41.*

33.   Hockenberry-Eaton, M. & Powell, M.L. (1991). Merging advanced practice roles: The NP and CNS. *Journal of Pediatric Health Care 5:158-159.*

34.   Kinlein, M.L. (1972). Independent nurse practitioner. *Nursing Outlook 20:22-24.*

35.   Mastrangelo, R. (1994). Be well and productive! *Advance for Nurse Practitioners 2(2): 17, 28.*

36.   Jacox, A.K. & Norris, C.M. (Eds.) (1977). *Organizing for Independent Nursing Practice.* New York: Appleton-Century-Crofts. pp. 2-6.

37.   Division of Nursing. (1994). Division defines the APN workforce. *American Journal of Nursing 94(10): 68, 70-71.*

38.   Hodnicki, D. (1988). Nurses—meeting the needs of the homeless. *Newsletter of the Council of Primary Health Care Nurse Practitioners 11(3):1.*

39.   Durham, J.D. & Hardin, S.B. (1985). Promoting advanced nursing practice. *The Nurse Practitioner 10(12):59-62.*

40.   Slattery, M. (1998, Nov./Dec.). Nurse-midwife empowers inner-city women through birth center. *The American Nurse, 11.*

41.   Wells, N., Johnson, R. & Salyer, S. (1998). Interdisciplinary collaboration. *Clinical Nurse Specialist 12(4):161-168.*

42.   Ball, G.B. (1990). Perspectives on developing, marketing, and implementing a new clinical nurse specialist position. *Clinical Nurse Specialist 4(1):33-36.*

43.   Towers, J. (1990). Report of the national survey of the American Academy of Nurse Practitioners, Part IV: Practice characteristics and marketing activities of nurse practitioners. *Journal of the American Academy of Nurse Practitioners 2(4):164-167.*

44.   Hershey, N (1980). A health lawyer's view. *Nursing Law and Ethics 1:1, 5.*

45.   Soehren, P.M. & Schumann, L.L. (1994). Enhanced role opportunities available to the CNS/nurse practitioner. *Clinical Nurse Specialist 8(3):123-127.*

46.   Boccuzzi, N.K. (1998). CAPNA. *American Journal of Nursing 98(11):34-35.*

47. Hester, L.E. & White, M.J. (1996). Perceptions of practicing CNSs about their future role. *Clinical Nurse Specialist 10(4):190-193.*
48. Moore, S.M. (1993). Promoting advanced practice nursing. *AACN Clinical Issues 4:603-608.*
49. Tucker, S., Sandvik, G., Clark, J., et al. (1999). Enhancing psychiatric nursing practice: Role of an advanced practice nurse. *Clinical Nurse Specialist 3(3):133-139.*
50. Towers, J. (1991). Report of the national survey of the American Academy of Nurse Practitioners, Part II: Pharmacologic management practices. *Journal of the American Academy of Nurse Practitioners 1(4):137.*
51. Burge, S., Crigler, L., Hurt, L., Kelly, G. & Sanborn, C. (1989). Clinical nurse specialist role development: Quantifying actual practice over three years. *Clinical Nurse Specialist 3(1):33-36.*4
52. Norwood, S.L. (1998). Psychiatric consultation liaison nursing: Revisiting the role. *Clinical Nurse Specialist 12(4):153-156.*
53. Picella, D.V. (1996). Use of a relational database program for quantification of the CNS role. *Clinical Nurse Specialist 10(6):301-308.*
54. Lund, S.M. (1994). Family-centered nurse coordinator—early childhood intervention: Development and implementation of the CNS role. *Clinical Nurse Specialist 8(2):109-113.*
55. Stimpson, M. & Hanley, B. (1991). Nurse policy analyst: Advanced practice role. *Nursing & Health Care 12(1):10-15.*
56. Berger, A.M., Eilers, J.G., Pattrin, L., et al. (1996). Advanced practice roles for nurses in tomorrow's health care systems. *Clinical Nurse Specialist 10(5):250-255.*
57. McFadden, E.A. & Miller, M.A. (1994). Clinical nurse specialist practice: Facilitators and barriers. *Clinical Nurse Specialist 8(1):27-33.*
58. Aikin, J.L., Taggart, J.R. & Tripoli, C.A. (1993). Evaluation and time documentation for the clinical nurse specialist. *Clinical Nurse Specialist 7(1):33-38.*
59. Fagin, C.M. (1977). Nature and scope of nursing practice in meeting primary health care needs. In: *Primary Care by Nurses: Sphere of Responsibility and Accountability.* Kansas City, MO: American Academy of Nursing. p. 39.
60. American Nurses' Association. *Nursing's Social Policy Statement.* (1995). 2nd ed. Washington, DC: ANA.
61. Styles, M.M. (1989). *On Specialization in Nursing: Toward a New Empowerment.* Kansas City, MO: American Nurses Foundation.
62. Riegel, B. & Murrell, T. (1987). Clinical nurse specialists in collaborative practice. *Clinical Nurse Specialist 1(2):63-69.*
63. *Nursing: A Social Policy Statement.* (1980). Kansas City, MO: American Nurses Association.
64. Mauksch, I.G. (1977). Unpublished speech given at Alpha Chi Chapter, Sigma Theta Tau, Boston College, MA., Feb. 28.
65. Mauksch, I.G. (1978). The nurse practitioner movement—where does it go from here? *American Journal of Public Health 68:1074-1075.*
66. Gardner, H.H. & Fiske, M.S. (1981). Pluralism and competition: A possibility

for primary care. *American Journal of Nursing 81:2152-2157.*

67.   Challela, M. (1979). The interdisciplinary team: A role definition for nursing. *Image 11:9-15.*

68.   Siegler, E.L. & Whitney, F.W. (1994). *Nurse-physician Collaboration: Care of Adults and the Elderly.* New York: Springer.

69.   Melvin, N. (1979). Developing guidelines for clinical privileges for nurse practitioners. In: *Power: Nursing's Challenge for Change.* Kansas City, MO: American Nurses' Association. p. 66.

70.   Siegler, E.L. & Whitney, F.W. (Eds.). *Nurse-physician Collaboration.* New York: Springer.

71.   Bates, B. (1972). Nurse-physician dyad: Collegial or competitive? In: *Three Challenges to the Nursing Profession.* New York: American Nurses' Association. p. 5.

72.   Sebas, M.B. (1994). Developing a collaborative practice agreement for the primary care setting. *Nurse Practitioner 19(3): 49-51.*

73.   Louis, M. & Sabo, C.E. (1994). Nurse practitioners: Need for and willingness to hire as viewed by nurse administrators, nurse practitioners, and physicians. *Journal of the American Academy of Nurse Practitioners 6:113-119.*

74.   Roueche, B. (Ed.) (1977). *Together: A Casebook of Joint Practices in Primary Care.* Chicago: The National Practice Commission. pp. vii, 2-16.

75.   Jacavone, J.B., Daniels,R.D., & Tyner, I. (1999). CNS facilitation of a cardiac surgery clinical pathway program. *Clinical Nurse Specialist 13(3):126-132.*

76.   Safriet, B.J. (1998). Still spending dollars, still searching for sense: Advance practice nursing in an era of regulatory and economic turmoil. *Advanced Practice Nursing Quarterly, 4(3):24-33.*

77.   Simmons, R.S. & Rosenthal, J. (1981). The women's movement and the nurse practitioner's sense of role. *Nursing Outlook 29:371-375.*

78.   Claiborn, S.A. & Walton, W. (1979). Pediatrician's acceptance of PNPs. *American Journal of Nursing 79:300.*

79.   Moses, E.B. (1993). Selected facts about nurse practitioners and nurse-midwives. *Fact Sheet.* Rockville, MD: Division of Nursing, Public Health Service, U.S. Department of Health and Human Services.

80.   Iglesias, G.H. (1998). Role evolution of the mental health clinical nurse specialist in home care. *Clinical Nurse Specialist 12(1):38-44.*

81.   Catlin, A.J. & McAuliffe, M. (1999). Proliferation of non-physician providers as reported in JAMA, 1998. *Image 31(2):175-177.*

82.   Page, N.E. & Arena, D.M. (1991). Practical strategies for CNS role implementation. *Clinical Nurse Specialist 5(1):43-48.*

83.   Moody, N.B., Smith, P.L. & Glenn, L.L. (1999). Client characteristics and practice patterns of nurse practitioners and physicians. *Nurse Practitioner 24(3):94-96, 99-100, 102-103.*

84.   Zwanziger, P.J., Peterson, R.M., Lethlean, H.M., et al. (1996). Expanding the CNS role to the community. *Clinical Nurse Specialist 10(4):199-202.*

85. Mundinger, M.O. (1994). Advanced-practice nursing—good medicine for physicians? *New England Journal of Medicine 330:211-213.*
86. Cohen, S.S., Meson, D.J., Arsenie, L.S.H., et al. (1998). Focus groups reveal perils and promises of managed care for nurse practitioners. *Nurse Practitioner, 23(6):48, 54, 57-58, 60, 63, 67-70, 76-77.*
87. Radke, K., McArt, E., Schmitt, M. & Walker, E.K. (1990). Administrative preparation of clinical nurse specialists. *Journal of Professional Nursing 6(4):221-228.*
88. O'Rourke, M.W. (1989). Generic professional behaviors: Implications for the clinical nurse specialist role. *Clinical Nurse Specialist 3(3):128-132.*
89. Booth, R.Z. (1995). Leadership challenges for nurse practitioner faculty. *Nurse Practitioner 20(4): 52-54, 56-58.*
90. Keenan, T. (1978). Birth of the fellowship program. In: *Nurse Faculty Fellowships in Primary Care.* Robert Wood Johnson Foundation, First Annual Symposium. pp. 22-23.
91. Minarik, P.A. (1990). Collaboration between service and education: Perils or pleasures for the clinical nurse specialist? *Clinical Nurse Specialist 4(2):109-114.*
92. Ryan-Merritt, M.V., Mitchell, C.A. & Pagel, I. (1988). Clinical nurse specialist role definition and operationalization. *Clinical Nurse Specialist 2(3):132-138.*
93. Knafl, K.A. (1978). How nurse practitioner students construct their role. *Nursing Outlook 26:650-653.*
94. Beare, P.G. (1989). The essentials of the win-win negotiation for the clinical nurse specialist. *Clinical Nurse Specialist 3(3):138-141.*
95. Van Fleet, S.K. (1996). Psychiatric CNS consultation model in a medical setting. *Clinical Nurse Specialist, 10(4):204-211.*
96. Hayes, E. (1994). Helping preceptors mentor the next generation of nurse practitioners. *Nurse Practitioner 19(6):62-66.*
97. Lukacs, J.L. (1982). Factors in nurse practitioner role adjustment. *The Nurse Practitioner 7:2-23, 50.*
98. Oda, D.S., Sparacino, P.S.A. & Boyd, P. (1988). Role advancement for the experienced clinical nurse specialist. *Clinical Nurse Specialist 2:167-171.*
99. Ford, L.C. (Nov. 13, 1980). Wellness: A focus for nursing practice. Unpublished paper presented at Wellness:Focus for the 80s. American Nurses' Association Annual Conference for the Council of Primary Health Care Nurse Practitioners. Philadelphia.
100. An interview with Dr. Loretta Ford. (1975). *The Nurse Practitioner 1:9-12.*
101. Mirr, M.P. (1993). Advanced clinical practice: A reconceptualized role. *AACN Clinical Issues 4:599-602.*
102. Nichols, L. (1992). Estimating costs of underusing advanced practice nurses. *Nursing Economics 10:343-351.*
103. Reading, B.A. (1994). Titling and the advanced practice nurse. *Advanced Practice Nurse, Spring/Summer, 7-8.*
104. Starck, P.L. (1995). Health care reform in '95: Six problems APNs must address. *American Journal of Nursing 95(1):16E-16F, 16H.*

105.   Kaufman, M., Hawkins, J.W., Higgins, L.P. & Friedman, A.H.. (1988). *Dictionary of American Nursing Biography.* Westport, CT: Greenwood.
106.   Bear, E.M. (1995). Advanced practice nurses: How did we get here anyway? *Advanced Practice Nursing Quarterly 1(1):10-14.*
107.   Keafer, M.R.. & Biester, D.J. (1993). Advanced practice in pediatric nursing. *Journal of Pediatric Nursing 8:263-264.*
108.   American Association of Colleges of Nursing. (1994). Position statement: Certification and regulation of advanced practice nurses. Washington DC.
109.   American Nurses Association (1993). Advanced practice nursing: A new age in health care. *Nursing Facts.* Washington DC: Author.
110.   Madden, M.J. & Ponte, P.R. (1992). Advanced practice roles in the managed care environment. *Journal of Nursing Administration 24(1):56-62.*
111.   American Nurses Association (1992). ¨Working definition: Nurses in advanced clinical practice. Washington DC: Author.
112.   National Task Force on Quality Nurse Practitioner Education. (1997). *Criteria for Evaluation of Nurse Practitioner Programs.* Washington, DC: National Organization of Nurse Practitioner Faculties.
113.   National Council of State Boards of Nursing. (1999). Model pharmacology/pharmacotherapeutics curriculum guidelines. Chicago:NCSBN.
114.   Miller, S.K. (1998). Defining the acute in acute care nurse practitioner. *Clinical Excellence for Nurse Practitioners 2(1):52-55.*
115.   Haines, J. (1992). *The nurse practitioner: A discussion paper.* Ottawa, Canada: Canadian Nurses Association.
116.   Wansborough, G. (1995, April). Nurse practitioner: CNO starts Extended Class application process. *Communique 18-19.*
117.   Wansborough, G. (1995, February). The Extended Class: Assessment and education program key to registration. *Communique 29-30.*
118.   Ministry of Health, Ontario. (1994). Nurse practitioners in Ontario: A plan for their education and employment. Ottawa, Ontario, Canada: Ministry of Health.
119.   Byrne, C., Bell, B., Roberts, J., et al. (1997). Primary care in Ontario, Canada: Implications for the complementary role of the nurse practitioner. *Clinical Excellence for Nurse Practitioners 1:15-21.*
120.   Chiarella, M. (1998). Independent, autonomous, or equal: What do we really want? *Clinical Excellence for Nurse Practitioners 2:293-299.*
121.   Peters, S. (1997, September). Blazing a trail in New Zealand: Getting to know Annette Milligan, BA, RCpN, FCNA. *Advance for Nurse Practitioners 57-58, 73.*
122.   Jones, M. (1997). Health care change and innovative practice in the United Kingdom. *Clinical Excellence for Nurse Practitioners 2:143-150.*
123.   Miller, D.S. & Backett, E.M. (1980). A new member of the team? Extending the role of the nurse in British primary care. *The Lancet 2:358-361.*
124.   Stillwell, B. (1984). The nurse in practice. *Nursing Mirror 158:17-22.*
125.   Zimmer, P.A. (1998). NPs in the Netherlands? Yes! An international conference—"Nurse practitioners challenging conventional roles in health

care." *Nurse Practitioner World News 3:1, 3, 8.*
126. Shvarts, S. & Frenkel, D.A. (1998). Nurses in Israel: The struggle for regulating the profession. *Clinical Excellence for Nurse Practitioners 2:376-382.*
127. Offredy, M. (1998). Nurse practitioners in the United Kingdom: Some considerations of the literature. *Clinical Excellence for Nurse Practitioners 2:307-313.*

BIBLIOGRAPHY

Abraham, T. & Fallon, P.J. (1997). Caring for the community: Development of the advanced practice nurse role. *Clinical Nurse Specialist 11:224-230.*

Brown, M.A. & Olshansky, E.E. (1997). From limbo to legitimacy: A theoretical model of the transition to the primary care nurse practitioner role. *Nursing Research 46:46-51.*

Brown, M.A. & Olshansky, E. (1998). Becoming a primary care nurse practitioner: Challenges of the initial year of practice. *Nurse Practitioner 23:46-66.*

Brush, B.L. & McGee, E.M. (1997). Revisiting 'a nurse for all settings': The nurse practitioner movement, 1965-1995. *Journal of the American Academy of Nurse Practitioners 8(1):5-11.*

Brush, B.L. & Capezuti, E.A. (1999). The expanded care for healthy outcomes (ECHO) project: Addressing the spiritual care needs of homeless men in recovery. *Clinical Excellence for Nurse Practitioners: The International Journal of NPACE 3(2):116-122.*

Cotton, A.H. (1997). Power, knowledge, and the discourse of specialization in nursing. *Clinical Nurse Specialist 11:25-29.*

Fine, S. (1997). *Developing a Private Practice in Psychiatric Mental-health Nursing.* New York: Springer.

Hamric, A.B., Spross, J.A. & Hanson, C. (1996). *Advanced Nursing Practice.* Philadelphia:Saunders.

Hawkins, J.W., Veeder, N.W. & Pearce, C.W. (1998). *Nurse-social Worker Collaboration in Managed Care: A Model of Community Case Management.* New York: Springer.

Kleinpell, R.M. & Piano, M.R. (Eds.) (1998). *Practice Issues for the Acute Care Nurse Practitioner.* New York:Springer.

Lasker, R.D. & the Committee on Medicine and Public Health. (1997). *Medicine & Public Health.* New York: The New York Academy of Medicine.

Mezey, M.D. & McGivern, D.O. (Eds.) (1999). Nurses, Nurse Practitioners: Evolution to Advanced Practice. 3rd ed. New York: Springer.

Miller, S.K. (1998). Defining the acute in acute care nurse practitioners. *Clinical Excellence for Nurse Practitioners 2:52-55.*

Schraeder, C., Lamb, G., Shelton, P. & Britt, T. (1997). Community nursing organizations: A new frontier. *American Journal of Nursing 97(1):63-65.*

Snyder, M. & Mirr, M.P. (1995). *Advanced Practice Nursing: A Guide to Professional Development.* New York: Springer.

Stotts, D.R., Rider, B. & Koster, B. (1997). A profile of West Virginia nurse prac-

titioners. *Clinical Excellence for Nurse Practitioners 1:444-448.*
Veeder, N.W. (1999). *Marketing Human Services: Selling Your Services under Managed Care.* New York: Springer.

ONLINE RESOURCES

Maxwell, B. (1998). *How to Find Health Information on the Internet.* Washington, D.C.: American Public Health Association.

See columns in every issue of *Clinical Excellence for Nurse Practitioners: The International Journal of NPACE, 1-4:1997-2000.*

Resource for all health care professionals: The Best Practice Network Website: **www.best4health.org**

Resources for NP students: **http://nurseweb.ucsf.edu/www/arwwebpg/htm**

NP Listserv: **www.son.washington.edu/npinfo/html**

NP nursing links (United Kingdom and United States): **www.healthcentre.org.uk/np/links/htm**

Nurse Practitioner Support Services (including national job search listings: **www.nurse.net/np/index2.html**

Nursing connection: **http://home.earthlink.net/~mjsevero**

PEW website: **www.futurehealth.ucsf.edu/pubs.html**

The Internet's nursing index: **www.wwnurse.com**

2

Using a Nursing Model for Advanced Practice

Introduction

The role of the advanced practitioner is multifaceted, complex and diversified. Inherent in the role is accountability and responsibility for decisions made and actions rendered. This responsibility is retained even when a referral to another health care provider is indicated. By using a nursing model as a guide, the advanced practice nurse can assess the supports and constraints within the system and plan care accordingly. Constraints can be identified and strategies can be developed to overcome them. Supports can be mobilized to provide high quality nursing care.

Nursing Models

A nursing model provides detailed guidelines for organizing and collecting data to be used for planning and implementing management and change strategies and evaluating total role functions. A model defines the essence and boundaries of the care rendered as well as explicitly stating the role of the nurse and the patient. Delineating boundaries is especially important in light of the legal ramifications associated with advanced practice and expanded role function. A nursing model also specifies the ultimate goal of the nursing process. This is an important aspect to clarify because the ultimate goal of the nursing process, as dictated by one's model of practice, may differ from that of the agency employing the practitioner or clinical specialist. This discrepancy can lead to basic philosophical differences which can cause role conflict and confusion. A nursing model helps to bring the often nebulous philosophical issues into sharper focus.

At the present time, there are many models of nursing practice in various stages of development. Among these are the Crisis Model, the Rogers Life Process Model, the Roy Adaptation Model, Orem's Self Care Model, King's Goal Attainment, and the Neuman Health Care Systems Model. Caring is the focus of a number of contemporary models. Among these are those of Benner and Wrubel, Leininger, and Watson. Advanced practice nurses must think carefully about their philosophies of nursing and health care and about the relationships between these two belief systems. Since one's philosophy is derived from one's cultural and social experiences, there is no right or wrong philosophy. One must honestly strive to know what one believes about nursing and its practice so that a model of practice can be chosen that is compatible with these beliefs. Thibodeau's *Nursing Models: Analysis and Evaluation* gives specific guidelines for selecting and evaluating a model of practice (1) (also see this chapter's bibliography).

Advanced clinical practice and expanded nursing role functions should be guided by a nursing model and not by the medical model. Nursing management of patients, patient advocacy, improvement of methods of health care delivery, and broad health assessment and planning are integral components of nursing's role. These functions are not extensions of medicine, nor do they fall within the framework of medical protocols.

In education, practice, and research, nursing has clearly been moving away from the medical model approach to health care delivery. A study by Thibodeau and Hawkins (2) found that advanced practitioners see themselves as nurses with a broader focus than that inherent in the medical paradigm. These nurses have strong images of themselves in their roles through their strong orientation toward a nursing model. Early nurse practitioner programs were directed or co-directed by physicians. As a result, there has always been the danger, particularly for these advanced practice nurses, of practicing according to the medical rather than a nursing model in the nurse's delivery of primary care. Incorporating physical assessment and history-taking skills into one's practice does not have to lead to junior doctoring. Nurses and physicians should complement each other because their assessment skills are utilized for different ends. The acute care setting, with its history of medical dominance, holds the same danger for the clinical nurse specialist of being co-opted by the medical model. So do the practices of nurse-midwives and nurse anesthetists. And *their* advanced practice specialties preceded the medical specialties!

The lure of following the medical model is sanctioned and well rewarded in some settings. Johnson (3) states that a number of nurses have chosen the medical model of practice because they do not think nursing has a destiny of its own or because they believe their identity depends on the sanction of physicians. Some nurses may feel that the medical model offers them greater challenges and responsibilities—until they realize that nurses can never have freedom and autonomy using that model.

The medical model focuses on signs, symptoms, pathology, prognoses, and the course of disease. This disease-oriented approach attends to the structure and functions of the body rather than to the total person. It ignores the environment and the psychosocial factors that surround illness, including quality of life and ethics (4). "The medical model posits a dichotomy between mind and body which is not congruent with the philosophy of nursing in its concerns with the whole person. Not only is nursing concerned with the structure and function of the body; it is also concerned with human experience, behavior, feelings, and the influence of social forces upon the body—manifestations of the man-environment interaction" (5). The nurse's advanced practice role in clinical practice should not have a medical orientation. Since assessment skills are used as adjuncts to the nursing process, their incorporation into the nursing role is best done within the context of a conceptual model of nursing practice.

What is the essence of nursing, its boundaries, and its goals? Although there is still much discussion as to the nature of nursing, there is basic agreement within the profession as to the four essential concepts of a nursing model. These are: person, environment, health, and nursing. Other disciplines may address one, two, or even three of these concepts, but all four elements must be addressed if a model is to be considered a nursing model.

Person. A nursing model must describe the nature of the person. The individual may be seen as an active or passive being who cooperated with the environment, controls the environment, or is controlled by it.

The wholeness and integrity of the individual may be emphasized, or emphasis may be placed on individual, unique attributes. Equal attention may be placed on the physical, spiritual, social, cultural, and psychological aspects of the individual's nature, or some aspects of the person may receive undue attention to the exclusion of other aspects. The nature of the person influences very directly the nature of nursing.

Environment. Environment can be viewed as all of the influences and circumstances surrounding and affecting people. Environment has both an internal and an external component. The internal environment relates to factors such as personality, mental capacity, and genetic make-up. The external environment includes all factors outside the individual. The nurse is part of the individual's external environment. It is evident that the nature of person-environment interactions as described by a given model also greatly influences the nature of nursing.

Health. Health and illness may be conceptualized on a continuum as co-existent states or mutually exclusive states (see Figure 1.1). Health may be viewed as a behavior or from a physical, mental or social perspective. A physical perspective emphasizes observable and measurable manifestations of illness. A mental perspective emphasizes the person's state of mind, that is, how the individual feels. A social perspective emphasizes disruptions in activities of daily living or inability to carry out prescribed roles, such as that of parent or worker. Health-illness is described in any given nursing model. Since one of the goals of nursing is to promote health, it is evident how the perception of health directly influences the practice of nursing.

Knutson (6) suggests that the evolution from a medical to a nursing model has changed the focus of our practices from illness care to health care.

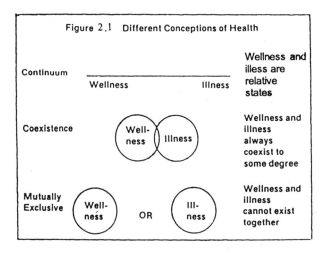

Figure 2.1 Different Conceptions of Health

Nursing. Nursing models speak specifically to the nature of nursing, its goals, and the process utilized to achieve these goals. The role of the nurse is implicitly or explicitly addressed in any given nursing model.

At the present time, there is no dominant model for nursing that clearly and explicitly guides the majority of practitioners of nursing. Nor does one model set the direction for all nursing education and research endeavors. Today, any nursing model only dictates that the four essential components of nursing's metaparadigm (person, health, environment, and nursing) be addressed. A nursing model describes how each of these elements is precisely defined and depicted. By doing so, it focuses thinking in a particular way. Wilbur (7) suggests that advanced practice nurses are developing their own theoretical frameworks out of their practice experiences. A model outlines nursing practice in a way that can be reality tested and corroborated. Nursing models are devices by which assumptions held by nurses about their practice can be transformed into postulates, which in turn can be tested through research.

A model generates researchable questions which, if answered by a process of scientific inquiry, lead to the development of nursing theory. This theory would truly belong to the field of nursing and could be described as unique rather than borrowed theory. Johnson describes borrowed theory as knowledge that is developed by other disciplines and is then drawn upon by nursing. Unique theory is that knowledge derived from generation of hypotheses unlike those that characterize other disciplines (8). A nursing model is the direct pathway to nursing theory.

Use of a Nursing Model in Advanced Practice
A model directly guides nursing management of patients in all health care settings. It guides the collection of data, the planning of care, the implementation of care, and the evaluation of that care. Since the model outlines the boundaries and essence of the discipline, practice of a given model is directly related to the scope of practice, practice-generated research, and quality of care. (See Chapters 1, 3 and 11.)

A Paradigm Shift for the New Millennium
Advanced nursing practice has evolved from ties with the medical model to a nursing paradigm which has generated several mid-range practice theories (e.g., pain, chronic illness, fatigue, caring and comfort measures, and family caregiver strategies) specific to the discipline of nursing (9, 10, 11, 12). This chapter has discussed the distinction between the medical model and the nursing model and how a model guides processes and determines outcomes.

Chapter 1 presented the historical evolution of advanced nursing practice. As we begin the new millennium we, in some ways, have come full circle from ancient practices to new age health care. Early uses of magnets, herbals, and homeopathic remedies are being re-examined in scientific studies. For example, a large, randomized multicentered clinical trial sponsored by the NIH is underway to test the efficacy of St. John's wort on depression (13). The role of prayer and spirituality in healing is also re-emerging.

The NIH has created an Office of Alternative Medicine (OAM) which is comprised of 7 sectors: mind-body interventions; bioelectrical therapies; alternative systems of medical practice (acupuncture and homeopathy); manual healing methods (chiropractic); pharmaceutical and biological therapies; herbal medicine and nutrition (14). The OAM works closely with the Food and Drug Administration (FDA) to advance clinical research and acceptance of alternative modalities, particularly acupuncture and botanicals. Joint efforts of the OAM and the FDA have affected the legal-regulatory arena and health policy such as the legalization of acupuncture needles in 1996. The FDA is currently drafting policy for the development of botanicals in the United States (13). Many major insurers are now covering and promoting the use of health and fitness clubs, nutritional counseling, and educational sessions to prevent problems and more effectively manage existing health problems.

Advanced practice nurses must be very cognizant of alternative therapies and assess how they complement nursing practice (15, 16). The findings of two large surveys in the United Kingdom and the United States indicate that nurses have incorporated (in order of frequency) message, aromatherapy, reflexology, relaxation, visualization, and acupuncture into their practices. These strategies were most frequently employed in community, hospice, and oncology settings (17, 18). A survey of over 600 primary care physicians and nurse practitioners found that 90% of physicians and practitioners report recommending at least one method of alternative therapy, primarily for pain management (19).

The concept of interdisciplinary collaboration must be expanded to include, for example, naturopaths, spiritual healers, and acupuncturists. The aggregate number of advanced nurse practitioners, physician assistants, midwives, chiropractors, acupuncturists, naturopaths, optometrists, and podiatrists doubled between 1992 and 1997 and a further increase of 20% is projected for 1001 (20).

Nursing histories must include cultural beliefs and alternative treatment and preventative strategies. Seventy percent of middle-aged adults and 50% of senior citizens are interested in having alternative therapies incorporated into their health care protocols (19). In 1998, a survey of Florida residents found 62% used alternative therapies, including relaxation techniques, herbal medicines, acupuncture, energy healing, and hypnosis (21). A study of 503 persons diagnosed with cancer indicated that 16% utilized alternative therapies and that 85% believed that alternative care should be offered at all cancer treatment centers (22).

Widespread use of the internet to access research and health care information and referrals, chat rooms with others experiencing similar health problems, proliferation of alternative health publications, health hotlines and outreach centers associated with health care institutions all contribute to more active, sophisticated consumers of health care.

In the new millennium, more than ever, the patient is an active partner in his or her health plan and any model used to guide practice must be grounded in that assumption. Eisenberg (23) proposed a strategy whereby health care providers and their patients proactively discuss preferences and expectations. The patients maintain symptom and quality of life diaries and determine the frequency and scheduling of follow-up visits with the health care provider.

Summary
A nursing model provides guidelines for the role functions of advanced practice nurses. The philosophy of the practitioner determines his or her choice of a model of nursing practice. One's model of practice has implications for all areas of role function, including standards of practice, legal-regulatory aspects, and continuous quality improvement.

REFERENCES

1. Thibodeau, J. (1983). *Nursing Models: Analysis and Evaluation*. Monterey, CA: Wadsworth.
2. Thibodeau, J. & Hawkins, J. (1994). Moving toward a nursing model in advanced practice. *Western Journal of Nursing Research 16(2):205-218*.

3. Johnson, P.E. (1974). Development of theory: A requisite for nursing as a primary health profession. *Nursing Research 23:372-377.*
4. Allen, J. & Hall, B. (1988). Changing the focus on technology: A critique of the medical model in the health care system. *Advances in Nursing Science 10:22-35.*
5. Phillips, J.R.(1977). Nursing systems and nursing models. *Image 9:4-7.*
6. Knutson, K. (1990). 25 years later: 25 exceptional NPs look at the movement's evolution and consider future challenges for the role. *The Nurse Practitioner 15:20.*
7. Wilbur, J. (1990). 25 years later: 25 exceptional NPs look at the movement's evolution and consider future challenges for the role. *The Nurse Practitioner 15:14.*
8. Johnson, P.E. (1968). Theory in nursing: Borrowed and unique. *Nursing Research 17:206-209.*
9. Dluhy, N.M. (1995). Mapping knowledge in chronic illness. *Journal of Advanced Nursing 21(6):1051-1058.*
10. Jenny, J. & Logan, J. (1996). Caring and comfort metaphors used by patients in critical care. *Image: Journal of Nursing Scholarship 28(4):349-252.*
11. Nolan, M. & Grant, G. (1992). Mid-range theory building and the nursing theory-practice gap: A respite care case study. *Journal of Advanced Nursing 17(2):217-223.*
12. Pierce, L.L. (1997). The framework of systemic organization applied to older adults as family caregivers of persons with chronic illness and disability. *Gastroenterology Nursing 20(5):168-175.*
13. Eskinazi, D. & Hoffman, F.A. (1998). Progress in complementary and alternative medicine: A contribution of the National Institutes of Health and the Food and Drug Administration. *Journal of Alternative and Complementary Medicine 4(4):459-467.*
14. Gordon, J.S. (1996). Alternative medicine and the family physician. *American Family Physician 52(7):2218-2220.*
15. Gates, B. (1994). The use of complementary and alternatives therapies in health care: A selective review of the literature and discussion of the implications for nurse practitioners and health-care managers. *Journal of Clinical Nursing 3(1):43-47.*
16. Teschendorff, J. & Chew, D. (1993). East meets west: Nurses learning complementary healing therapies. *Australian Nurses Journal 22(9):16-19.*
17. Rankin-Box, D. (1997). Therapies in practice: A survey assessing nurses' use of complementary therapies. *Complementary Therapy Nurse Midwifery 3(3):92-99.*
18. Wearn, A.M. & Greenfield, S.M. (1998). Access to complementary medicine in general practice: Survey in one UK health authority. *Journal of Society and Medicine 91(9):465-470.*
19. Gordon, N.P. & Sobel, D.S. (1998). Use of and interest in alternative therapies among adult primary care clinicians and adult members in a large health maintenance organization. *Western Journal of Medicine 169(3):153-161.*
20. Cooper, R.A. & Laud, P. (1998). Current and projected workforce of

nonphysician clinicians. *Journal of the American Medical Association 280(9):788-794.*
21. Burg, M.A. & Hatch, R.L. (1998). Lifetime use of alternative therapy: A study of Florida residents. *Southern Medical Journal 91(12):1126-1131.*
22. Coss, R. & McGrath, P. (1998). Alternative care. Patient choices for adjunct therapies within a cancer center. *Cancer Practitioner 6(3):176-181.*
23. Eisenberg, D.M. (1997). Advising patients who seek alternative medical therapies. *Annals of Internal Medicine 127(1):61-69.*

BIBLIOGRAPHY

Benner, P. & Wrubel, J. (1989). *The Primacy of Caring.* Menlo Park, CA:Addison-Wesley.
Chinn, P.S. & Krammer, M. (1995). *Theory and Nursing: A Systematic Approach.* (4th ed.) St. Louis, MO: Mosby-Yearbook.
Clark, C.C., Gordon, R., Harris, B. & Helvie, C.O. (1999). *Encyclopedia of Complementary Health Practice.* New York:Springer.
Copnell, B. (1998). Synthesis in nursing knowledge: An analysis of two approaches. *Journal of Advanced Nursing 27(4):870-874.*
Daniels, G.J. & McCabe, P. (1994). Nursing diagnosis and natural therapies: A symbiotic relationship. *Journal of Holistic Nursing 12(2):184-192.*
Gordon, R.J., Nienstedt, B.C. & Gesler, W.M., eds. (1998). *Alternative Therapies.* New York:Springer.
Fawcett, J. (1993). *Analysis and Evaluation of Nursing Theories.* Philadelphia: F.A. Davis.
Hampton, D. (1994). King's theory of goal attainment as a framework for managed care implementation in a hospital setting. *Nursing Science Quarterly 7:170-173.*
Hatgidakis, J.E. & Timko, E.R. (1997). Spirituality and practice. Stories, barriers, and opportunities. *Creativity in Nursing 3(4):7-11.*
Hawkins, J., Thibodeau, J., Utley-Smith, Q.E., Igou, J.F. & Johnson, E.E. (1993). Using a conceptual model for practice in a nursing wellness center for seniors. *Perspectives: Journal of the Gerontological Nursing Association l7(4):11-16.*
Hawkins, J. & Thibodeau, J. (1994). 25+ and going strong: Nurse practitioners and and nursing practice. *Journal of the American Academy of Nurse Practitioners 11:525-531.*
Kenney, J.W. (1999). *Philosophical and Theoretical Perspectives for Advanced Nurse Practice.* (2nd ed.) Sudbury, MA: Jones & Bartlett.
Leininger, M. (1991). *Culture Care Diversity and Universality: A Theory of Nursing.* New York: National League for Nursing.
Lutz, K.F. & Jones, K.D. (1997). Expanding the praxis debate: Contributions to clinical inquiry. *Advances in Nursing Science 20(2):23-31.*
Marriner-Tomey, A. (1994). *Nursing Theorists and Their Work.* 3rd ed. St. Louis, MO: C.V. Mosby.
Meleis, A. (1997). *Theoretical Nursing: Development and Progress.* Philadelphia: Lippincott.

Nagle, L.M. & Ryan, S.A. (1996). The superhighway to nursing science and practice. *Holistic Nursing Practice 1(1):25-30.*

Neuman, B. (1988). *The Neuman Systems Model.* Norwalk, CT: Appleton & Lange.

Newman, M.A. (1994). *Health as Expanding Consciousness.* 2nd ed. New York: National League for Nursing.

Orem, D.E. (1985). *Concepts of Practice.* 3rd ed. New York: McGraw-Hill.

Rankin-Box, D.F. (1996). Is there a place for complementary therapies in the accident and emergency department? *Accident and Emergency Nursing 4(3): 160-164.*

Rogers, M. (1985). *An Introduction to the Theoretical Basis of Nursing.* Philadelphia: F.A. Davis.

Roy, Sr.C. & Andrews, H.A. (1991). *Roy Adaptation Model.* Norwalk, CT: Appleton & Lange.

Snyder, M. & Lindquist, R., eds. (1998). *Complementary/Alternative Therapies in Nursing.* New York:Springer.

Vander Henst, J.A. (1997). Client empowerment: A nursing challenge. *Clinical Nurse Specialist 11(3):96-99.*

Walker, L.O. & Avant, K. (1995). *Strategies for Theory Construction.* (3rd ed.) Norwalk, CT:Appleton & Lange.

Watson, J. (1995). Nursing's caring-healing paradigm as an exemplar for alternative medicine? *Alternative Therapies in Health & Medicine 1(3):64-69.*

Watson, J. (1994). *Applying the Art and Science of Human Caring.* New York: National League for Nursing.

Watson, J. (1988). *Nursing: Human Science and Human Care.* New York: National League for Nursing.

Woolery, L. & Yensen, J. (1995). Nursing collaboratory development via the internet. *Medinfo 8(2):1349-1352.*

3

The Role of Research in Advanced Practice

Introduction

Research should be an integral part of the advanced practitioner's role. First, if nursing is to continue to move toward a more influential position concerning health care policy and delivery, we will need to demonstrate competence in knowledge and action. Second, if nurses are to justify their roles as providers within the health care delivery system, we are going to have to document that what we do for patients makes a difference. Escalating costs and changes in health care delivery venues dictate the need for professional accountability. To be accountable, we must be able to document "measurable change in health status and quality of life" (1, p. 190) Research is the means by which outcomes can be validated, the value of nursing management demonstrated, and our practice quantified as unique and, in some cases, superior to that of other health care professionals. Since we compete, in part, for a market of patients, we must be able to document what we have to offer them.

Since not all advanced practice nurses have the skills to conduct research, levels of participation must necessarily vary. Participants in research can be subjects, research assistants, consultants on content and nursing aspects, or principal investigators for a project (2, 67). In addition, all nurses in advanced practice can become knowledgeable consumers of research and assist other nurses to critique research findings for application in their practice (55).

Historical Background

Prior to 1952, a total of 259 nursing articles can be identified as having a basis in research. Most of these dealt with issues of nursing function, welfare, curriculum, and procedures. Only a few clinical research articles appeared, mostly in the area of maternal-child health. Of the authors of these articles, only 60% were nurses (3). The inventory of nurses published by the ANA represented the first systematic attempt at data collection about the profession. Yet, as early as 1949, Esther Lucile Brown identified research as a component of the nursing role (4), and in 1950, the National League for Nursing Publication Conference emphasized the need for research to help students solve problems (3).

The first issue of *Nursing Research* was published in June 1952. That was also the year in which the Joint Committee on Nursing Research and Studies published its philosophy and Plan of Action (6). In the following year, the Institute of Research and Service in Nursing Education was established at Teachers College, Columbia University, and Virginia Henderson of Yale's School of Nursing and Leo Simmons, a member of Yale's Sociology Department, began a survey and assessment of nursing research (3). Such was the growth of the movement that at the 1960 ANA convention over 800 nurses attended the Research Conference Group (3).

In 1965, the first nursing conference dedicated to research was held under the joint sponsorship of the American Nurses Association and the American Nurses Foundation, the latter with origins dating to the 1950 ANA series of studies on the functions of nursing (3).

Early publications on nursing research include *Nursing Research: Survey and Assessment* by Simmons and Henderson, 1964 (7), *Fundamentals of Research in Nursing* by Fox, 1966 (8), and *Better Patient Care through Nursing Research* by Abdellah and Levine, 1965 (9). The ANA convention in 1974 witnessed the presentation of two research papers to standing-room-only crowds. Of particular importance is that both papers focused on clinical nursing concerns and their relationship to research.

Thus, nursing research had, by 1976, to quote Elizabeth Carnegie, "Come of age within the past 25 years" (3, p. 23). The number of nurses prepared at the master's level has grown from only a few in the late twenties to an estimated more than 9% of the nursing work force in 1999 (11). Impetus has been added over the past three and a half decades by the availability of federal nurse traineeship monies to support preparation of nurses at the master's and doctoral levels and the creation of the National Center for Nursing Research that became, in 1993, the National Institute for Nursing Research (10).

Advanced Practice Research Today

Because of the importance of research to practice and to the role of the nurse in advanced practice, it is important for those without research skills to acquire them by continuing their formal education and by participating, at some level, in the research process.

Jacox and Norris have written that "the need for careful research designed to answer relevant questions is paramount for the nurse practitioner movement" (12). They could have been referring to all advanced practice nurses. Nurses practice as care providers in settings unfamiliar to physicians, such as in homes and other community settings and in geographic areas where there are no physicians. The populations they serve may be the poor, the aged, or minorities. Nurses focus on health care and on return to optimal level of functioning and not on curing illnesses, although they may be involved in illness care. They utilize management strategies that incorporate self-care, health education, and collaboration with patients. They assist patients to adapt to limitations. All of these facets of nursing practice need to be researched in order to strengthen the power base of nurses in advanced practice. We need also to explore health and illness behaviors and measure outcomes of nursing management strategies on these as well as on pathological states (13, 43).

Barnard emphasizes the need for practitioners to collaborate in the entire research process (14). While Barnard uses the term practitioner in a broad sense, the message is certainly applicable to nurses engaged in advanced practice roles.

Research has a number of important contributions to make beyond affecting and enhancing the quality of care and promoting health. It provides an avenue for introducing innovations and change in practice and of being proactive in the face of the current chaos (59). It lends credibility to lobbying processes by providing data to support legislation on issues such as direct third-party reimbursement for care given by advanced practice nurses (12, 60). Research can be used to identify communities of underserved patients and to document their health care needs, to answer clinical questions, provide data for practice guidelines or protocols, evaluate care, and build the knowledge base for practice (1, 18, 19, 22, 61).

Identifying Researchable Problems
The first step in the research process is to identify researchable problems for nursing (15, 16). While it is not within the scope of this book to teach the research process, it seems pertinent to single out this step within the context of advanced practice. (See bibliography at end of chapter). The rapid growth of nursing's entry into primary care and case management has raised many important questions about advanced practice roles.

Research questions often flow from clinical practice issues. For example, noting that persons in a schizophrenia treatment program tended to gain weight as a side effect on medications, an advanced practice nurse was instrumental in the initiation of a study to investigate strategies to ameliorate this problem (41). Nurse-midwives and nurse practitioners in two different comprehensive prenatal care programs believed that their patients' outcomes were better than those of other women delivered at the same institutions. Together with faculty and their graduate students preparing for advanced practice roles, they designed a study to examine perinatal outcomes. Noting that the caesarean section rate for her adolescent patients seemed to be lower than the institution's rate, a nurse practitioner collaborated with a graduate student to examine the reason for this. A nurse anesthetist suspected that the effects of general anesthesia do not clear patients' bodies for many hours, if not days or weeks. If so, this would have implications for patients resuming normal activities after day surgery or even a brief hospital stay, particularly for safe driving and critical thinking. Acting on her suspicions, she designed a study to measure physiologic and behavioral sequelae of commonly used general anesthetic agents. Recognizing that women with breast cancer are surviving longer, a nurse practitioner and a clinical nurse specialist colleague designed a phenomenological study to learn about women who are long-term survivors (58).

The advent of computerized data bases in clinical settings makes data retrieval for quantitative studies much easier than paper and pencil retrieval or even entering data on computer from patient records. When patient care data are recorded on computerized records, it is possible to ask all sorts of questions of the data and to track outcomes of care. Collecting data is something advanced practice nurses do every day in practice. Those data, particularly if they are computerized, are available to ask clinical question of. Issues of protection of human subjects and of confidentiality of data must, of course, be addressed, but appropriate approval by the institutional review board or human subjects committee can be sought and consent forms for use of data integrated into caregiving, as needed. (18, 47, 48, 49.)

Financing of care by nurses is a critical issue, particularly in this time of spiralling health costs. In the aftermath of the growth of clinical specialist programs since 1954 and of nurse practitioner programs since 1965, it is important to step back and examine the fit between these educational programs and the needs of society. The same applies to programs preparing nurse-midwives and nurse anesthetists.

There is a need to examine the interface between advanced practice nurses with other professionals, including nurses (17). Studies of the unique contributions nursing can make to patient care and of the importance of nursing to health care delivery are needed (57). The experience a patient has with a nurse in advanced practice may be an important variable in the patient's choice of provider. Advanced practice nurses must demonstrate the benefits of their management if they expect to be reimbursed for it (1). Data are needed to hold nursing's own in the political arena and to support its positions in developing public policy for health care provision (34). Advanced practice nurses increasingly are expected to incorporate research activities into their roles. Cronenwett has written a succinct and useful guide to fulfilling that expectation, and other authors have addressed this component of the advanced practice nurse's role (1, 20, 21, 41, 50, 51, 52, 53). Collaboration between advanced practice nurses and nursing faculty can be one way to fulfill this expectation (23, 24, 25, 52). A number of broad issues for research readily suggest themselves: the fit between educational preparation and role expectations; role development and role performance after completion of a master's program; characteristics of practice settings and patient populations; the experiences of patients with selected health problems; and intervention and outcome studies with selected patient groups.

Put another way, nurses in advanced practice need to study issues of role definition, their credibility as providers of care, the politics of health care delivery, and the ethical issues surrounding the delivery of care. The controversies concerning educational preparation for new roles and functions need to be explored. There is a need to define research for nursing practice; to address the ethical issues involved in human subjects research; to inspect the progress of the state of the art in research within our profession; and to establish guidelines for educational preparation for nurse researchers.

Incorporating the Role of Researcher into Practice
A critical issue for nurses in advanced roles is finding the time to do research. The many demands on a nurse's time often preclude research as an integral part of practice. Research is pushed to the back burner and the someday that it will be undertaken never arrives. A mentoring relationship can foster research, as can an institutional commitment to research as an integral part of the role of the advanced practice nurse (33). Advanced practice nurses also have a role to play in facilitating research (23).

The major impediment to incorporating research into the nursing role is the belief that research is somehow separate and magical. Yet each of us in our everyday practice collects reams of data. Collaborative projects with other providers may be possible utilizing these data. It is also sometimes feasible to combine research and demonstration programs. The initiation of a new format for delivering services or establishing a demonstration project can provide the impetus for research (27).

Developing and implementing a role (such as that of nurse practitioner, clinical specialist, nurse-midwife, or nurse anesthetist) within an agency can generate research questions. The daily statistical records on patients seen, the problems they present, and the management strategies used provide a wealth of data. The development, implementation, and evaluation of protocols for nursing management may be necessary for practice within a particular state or institution (68). The product of this process—outcomes for patients—could be the subject of a piece of nursing research.

Cluster studies might be possible within an agency, perhaps with collaboration between providers and faculty utilizing the agency for student experiences. Service agencies need to develop clinical research programs and to involve their staff in research (41). Advanced practice nurses may be ideal coordinators for clinical drug trials (62). Several collaborative models have been developed and show promise for replication in other agencies and institutions (27, 28).

Some practical suggestions for integrating research into the role responsibilities of busy advanced practice nurses come from the literature and from clinical practice sites. A key to success is commitment to research as an important component of professional practice by administrators in large institutions or by members of the practice setting in small agencies (53). Expectations that research has the lowest priority, especially in very busy and cost-conscious delivery systems, are not always borne out. We know of one very busy community hospital-based clinic and a community health center in the same city where the commitment to research is very high. Staff members, including clerical and record room personnel, have been extremely cooperative and interested through several projects. In the community health center, the shared interest of an advanced practice nurse and a physician led to the formation of an ad hoc research group. Their commitment to research and willingness to be active participants and collaborators, as well as to undertake their own studies to answer clinical questions, exceeds that of most, if not all, the big teaching institutions in the state.

One author suggests several ways to integrate this role component (41). Addressing clinical problems through research in order to change practice is one motivator since change is easier to accomplish from a knowledge base (64). Establishing a program for using research findings is another approach (5, 55). The excitement of the dissemination part of the research process motivates some nurses to complete projects (56). Offering all nurses on a unit or in a setting the opportunity to participate in a project not only provides more hands to get the work done but also generates enthusiasm and energy (41). For multisite projects, research site coordinators (usually advanced practice nurses) can keep all participants informed and enthusiastic about the project (53).

Establishing a research group or network for nurses (63) with similar interests is a wonderful way to undertake a project. Where individuals might not complete projects alone, they are less likely to let colleagues down by not fulfilling their responsibilities to the group. Group energy and knowledge offsets individual feelings of inadequacy. Someone in the group is likely to be strong in design, another in statistics, and so on. In one investigation of nurses' interest in research, nurse characteristics were found to be the most important variables related to involvement in research (51). Working in a group helps to overcome individual characteristics that mediate against completion of a project.

Krywanio suggests that clinicians invite nurses in the academy as consultants or collaborators (52). The superior clinical skills of the full-time practitioner can complement the research skills of the academic nurse. Graduate students often look for research projects and have the time and motivation to assist with many study tasks.

Sometimes research is sponsored by a group outside a practice setting. A specialty organization, such as the American Association of Critical-Care Nurses (54), might sponsor a research project. Health care industries often look for agency collaborators. Some projects, such as one on decubitus ulcers for example, involve important nursing problems (50).

Making time for research is not easy. But it is essential if advanced practice nurses are to have a place in today's competitive and chaotic health care marketplace. Documenting what we do for patients, why the activities are essential to the well being of patients, and that care is cost effective is critical to survival as caregivers (1).

Funding for Research
Research can be costly if it involves materials, equipment, and time over and above those that are part of the service role of the provider or institution. Access to computer services for data retrieval, storage, analysis, and literature searches may also be necessary and will be an expense if such services are not approved or supported by the institution. Thus, soliciting support for research outside of the employing agency or, for the independent practitioner, outside of her or his own funds, may be necessary, and a grant may need to be applied for. Some institutions and agencies give small grants to support research. So do many professional organizations and specialty groups. (See Appendix E.)

Resources to help you write a grant for funding are included in this chapter's bibliography. Many professional organizations have funding research as part of their mission. Organizations for advanced practice nurses appear in Appendix G. Courses on grant writing are useful and so is eliciting help from someone who has written a successful grant.

Impediments to Research
In general, women have not been socialized into roles as thinkers, analyzers, and questioners. Additionally, women must often surmount difficulties not encountered by their male colleagues. The

average working woman puts in 80 hours a week; the average man puts in 50 hours. Children and/or household responsibilities, or other caregiving such as for elders, often are distractors. Women thus must be creative in order to be creative.

The orderly nature of nursing can stifle creativity also, for nurses are educated to be neat and compliant, assets that may be impediments in the research process according to Notter (26). Nurses are often trapped into believing that research must be quantitative and abstract, whereas action research (research which is incorporated into practice) may be more appropriate to the questions that must be answered to validate our practice. Qualitative methods may be more appropriate to some research questions we wish to answer.

We need to continue to move away from the medical model and generate and use our own models for research (26). Nurses have been characterized as doers rather than thinkers and we need to divest ourselves of that image. We need to focus on defining nursing and nursing's role. More replication studies are needed to advance nursing science (26). We have depended too long on research generated through master's theses and doctoral dissertations—we need more post-doctoral research and studies over time. Finally, we need to fully incorporate the role of researcher into our image of nursing. If we continue to view it as an awkward appendage, an honor reserved for a chosen few, or as an albatross hung around our necks by some zealous dean, department head, or administrator, we will continue to view research as just another demand on our time (65).

Incorporating Research Findings into Practice

"The translation of research is a responsibility of practitioners" (28). Embracing research as an integral part of the role of the nurse in advanced practice means not only involvement in conducting research, but also being an intelligent consumer of the research generated by others. Sometimes lack of knowledge about nursing research findings and inaccessible literature are barriers (65). Barnard (14) states that the key to this is getting researchers to interact with clinicians. A survey of nurses in New York State disclosed that one of the obstacles to applying research findings was obtaining these findings. The most frequently read nursing journals are those that contain the smallest number of research studies, according to Miller and Messinger (29), and this is borne out by recent data indicating that the journal with the largest number of readers publishes few, if any, research studies.

Conferences, staff development programs, and the distribution of summaries of research findings were cited as other sources of information in addition to journal articles (29). Incorporating into basic nursing education programs the skills of reading and critiquing research intelligently will accelerate the utilization of research findings (5). So will the inclusion of a research component in programs designed to prepare nurses for advanced practice roles.

One model for disseminating research findings to staff nurses has evolved. This was a deliberate and systematic plan built into the research process to identify and reach a larger population of nurses in practice, and was developed to expedite communication from researcher to practitioners. In this model, the findings were translated and evaluated (30). This represents one step forward in closing the gap between researchers and those in nursing who care directly for patients. Nurses in advanced practice can serve as facilitators for research utilization (31).

Exploring utilization of research among nurses in advanced practice is important to increasing their roles in facilitating utilization by others (32). A barrier to incorporating research findings into practice is nurses' self-image (16). Nurses do not always see themselves as capable of shaping their own practice. Exposure to research findings and evaluation of these findings for their implications for practice will encourage research use (16). Skills in using research are also necessary if research is to be applied to practice (35). The closer researchers and practitioners move together, the more relevant research will be to the problems practitioners encounter in their management of patient care and the more likely that the results of nursing research will effect change in practice (66).

Publishing

If research findings are to be applied in practice, they must be widely disseminated to those in practice. Thus, the publication of management strategies, protocols, case studies, and other data generated through practice and research can contribute to the body of knowledge about health care as delivered by nurses.

Why publish? Styles (36) has written that "the primary reason to publish is because the future of the profession depends on it." The profession needs to have evidence of its scholarship through publication. Then, too, there is the personal thrill of seeing one's work in print, of being recognized as an author, and of receiving the professional rewards accorded to published authors (36).

The first hurdle to cross in writing for publication is fear. We are tempted to wallow in the mire of fear of publishing. Our procrastination strategies would win prizes for creativity. In desperation, we retreat to the old cliche, "Oh, I can't write." If you can talk, you can write and, as a nurse, you probably do a lot of both every day.

Start small if you feel you won't have enough to say for an article or if the thought of 10 to 15 pages is overwhelming. Write a letter to the editor. Co-author your first writing effort (37). Both of these techniques help to overcome fear.

Another step in overcoming fear is to read. Critique the articles you read. Ask yourself, "Could I have written that?" "Could I have done better?" "Did the opening paragraph invite me to read further?"

Write about what you know. In preparing a manuscript for publication on a research project, think of your audience. They will want to know who, what, where, how, and why, and, most importantly, the implications of your article or book for their practice. Emphasize how you have incorporated the research process into your practice (if you have), cite related studies, and document accurately. It is frustrating to track down an incorrectly cited reference.

The steps in writing are similar to those in nursing process. First, assess your practice and your strengths as a nurse in advanced practice. Write about protocols or management strategies you have developed. If you have completed a research project, evaluate the outcomes for possible articles. What would you most like to share from your experience or your research? The arguments for or against selecting a refereed journal are many. A refereed journal is one which utilizes the opinions of three or more experts in the field who review a manuscript so that the journal's editor can decide whether to publish it. To eliminate bias, these are generally independent and blind reviews. A list of the referee status of nursing journals is available (38). The value of the opinions of experts in the field is that the editor benefits from diverse points of view (39). The reviews also allow for a submitted article to be judged against the body of substantive knowledge specific to the discipline (40). Conversely, it can be argued that the review panel can turn into "The Establishment" (40). The debate has no clear solution (38). To select a refereed versus a non-refereed journal must be an individual decision. Most important is selecting a journal that publishes articles of the type you wish to write.

Peruse journals in the field and select one which seems appropriate to the topic you have in mind. After selecting one, check it concerning article length, number of manuscript copies to submit, and other information pertinent to authors (38). This information is usually found on the page with the table of contents and publisher's information. You can also write to the editor and request information. A comparison of 92 journals was published in 1991 with respect to this type of information (38).

Plan your article. Research the topic in the literature or gather together the material from your study and organize it into subgroups. You may want to develop a detailed outline and work from that. It is useful to have on hand reference works that will give you information on preparing your manuscript. A list of suggested references on or related to writing is included in this chapter's bibliography.

If you plan to include tables or graphs, lay them out so they can be typed or reproduced easily. Avoid "alphabet soup" by spelling out all but the most obvious terms. Keep tables brief and uncluttered. Try to convey only the most important information and leave out unnecessary details peripheral to the main ideas or findings.

Photographs should be clear, glossy, and black and white. Photos are expensive to reproduce, so use only those essential to the message of your article. Line drawings (not shaded), on the other hand, involve no extra printing expense. Often journals will assist you by providing photographs or line drawings if they will enhance the article. Sources of photographs run the gamut from those you or your colleagues take, to professional medical photographers, to archives. A computer makes sophisticated graphics and tables possible.

A writer's workshop can be helpful, particularly for the beginner. A workshop is generally designed to assist those who are novices to develop their ideas and carry them through to the point of submission to a journal. The format is usually informal and involves the active participation of those attending. Group support is a side benefit. A workshop can also help prepare the potential writer with some of the basic ingredients: how to write a query letter or an outline, and how to overcome some of the first-time jitters about the review process.

In the end, "a workshop is no substitute for writing and writing and *writing"* (43). Making time to write is important. Some helpful hints for advanced practice nurses appeared in a professional newsletter (44). Set aside a block of time and use it only for writing. Since time will not make itself, you will have to make time to write.

Finally, when there is no way out, sit down and write. Don't worry about writing in sequence. If the introduction just won't come, begin to write the part that seems easiest. Set short-term goals and reward yourself when goals are attained. Write in a straightforward manner and use the active voice whenever possible. Avoid sounding pedantic or pompous. Double-check all figures, totals, and tables, and use up-to date information (42). Most of all, keep writing.

An evaluation of the product of your efforts can take several forms. Solicit peer review by asking your colleagues to read what you have written and offer suggestions. If the material is clear to them, you have made your points well. If questions arise when they read your manuscript, incorporate the answers in your rewrite. If grammar is not your strong point, use one of the standard style manuals and seek out a reviewer who has skills in English. After the first draft, set your manuscript aside for a few days, then go back and reread it and see if it says what you mean to convey.

Follow your potential publisher's specifications for typing, style of documentation, margins, etc., precisely. A well-organized, neat manuscript makes a favorable impression. If you do not type well, have someone type for you. Using a word processor or computer is ideal. Proofread and correct carefully. Send the manuscript with the requested number of copies and include any supplementary material specified by the journal such as a black and white photograph of yourself, a brief biographical sketch, an abstract, and a curriculum vitae. Include your name, address, telephone number, job title, and affiliation. Write a brief, to-the-point letter to accompany the manuscript. Mail the manuscript in a padded mailer or sturdy manilla envelope. It is best to send it certified with a return receipt requested.

After you have mailed the manuscript, the waiting begins. Turnaround time for review varies widely. Check the information given by the journal you have submitted the manuscript to for an idea of when to expect a response. Most editors will acknowledge receipt, or your return receipt card will verify that the manuscript reached its destination. The review process is described in an excellent article by Swanson and McCloskey (45).

Major reasons for rejection include: subject already covered in a scheduled issue; subject too technical, inaccurate or undocumented; poor research design; faulty methodology; nursing aspects not well described; content unimportant; you have tried to convert a speech into an article; the conclusion is unwarranted by the data; the material has been published elsewhere; or the material is poorly presented (45). Some editors will write and give you a critique of the manuscript, whereas from others you will receive only a form letter or a polite thank you and please try again. Occasionally, rejection letters can be somewhat demoralizing, so develop a thick skin, learn from any helpful comments you can glean, reread and rewrite if necessary, and try again. Hints on handling rejection are included in a very useful article by two seasoned writers (46).

Other Ways of Disseminating Research Findings

Publishing is only one way of disseminating the results of a research project. Presenting research at a local, regional, or national meeting of a professional organization is another. Findings can be presented as a poster or as an oral research presentation. The first step is to respond to a call for abstracts. These can be found in professional journals and newsletters and often are distributed through flyers announcing a professional meeting and soliciting abstracts. Health care agencies and institutions and universities also sponsor research days and often include paper and poster presentations.

Abstracts. An abstract is an abbreviated version of your study, a summary. A typical abstract includes information about the background for the study, methods used, subjects, findings, conclusions, and recommendations, all in 100 to 500 words. It is important to follow the guidelines for submission of an abstract closely—use the form included in the directions, or the format requested, such as number of words, types of headings to use, single or double spacing, and so on. Typically, abstracts are reviewed blindly so you will probably be asked to provide a cover sheet listing your credentials and those of the other investigators, or a copy of the abstract with this information and several copies without it. The call for abstracts should specify whether the presentations will be oral or posters or both. You may be given a choice. Guidelines for preparing abstracts, oral presentations, and posters appear in this chapter's bibliography.

Posters. Posters can be free-standing or appropriate for an easel, a bulletin board, or a table top. Most conferences have guidelines as to what will be provided (an easel, bulletin board, or table) and what size and type to make your poster. If there are no directions, call and inquire of the conference organizers. There are commercial poster display units available and you may be able to borrow one from your agency, institution, or a professional organization. With computers, it is possible to prepare professional-looking posters yourself or pay a graphic artist to do so. A typical poster presentation format is to have an area set aside for posters and an allocated period of time for conference attendees to view them. You will sit or stand by your

poster and talk with attendees as they walk by.
Oral Presentations. An oral presentation of research is typically 10 to 30 minutes long. You will be given this information when your abstract is accepted for presentation or in the call for abstracts. The rule of thumb is two minutes per typed double-spaced page and no more than two slides per page. You can prepare your presentation from a typed script or present from narrative and data slides. Slide preparation has become simpler and cheaper through computer programs. Practice your presentation and time it carefully. It is helpful to have a colleague listen and critique your presentation. One of the most common problems new presenters have is time. Many conferences run on a very tight schedule and you may not be allowed to continue past your allocated time.

Presenting your research is an exciting culmination to a research project (56). It also helps build presentation skills, an important part of the role of the advanced practice nurse, and gives you an opportunity to talk with others who might be interested in the same topic or in applying your findings in their practice.

Summary
Research should not be neglected by nurses in advanced practice roles. As mavericks and risk takers in nursing, they can be leaders in clinical research as well. The field of nursing is so fertile that a rich harvest can be gleaned from the bounty of everyday practice in terms of researchable topics and issues that affect and shape the course of health care now and will affect and shape it in the future. Research will provide a sound rationale for what nurses in advanced practice roles do and what they say they do.

REFERENCES

1. Buchanan, L.M. (1994). Therapeutic nursing intervention: Knowledge development and outcome measures for advanced practice. *Nursing and Health Care 15:190-195.*
2. American Nurses Association. (1987). *Research in Nursing: Toward a Science of Nursing.* Kansas City, MO: Author.

3. Carnegie, M.E. (1976). *Historical Perspectives of Nursing Research.* Boston, MA: Boston University Mugar Memorial Library Nursing Archives. pp. 1-14.
4. Brown, E.L. (1949). *Nursing for the Future.* New York: Russell Sage. p. 100.
5. Stetler, C.B. (1994). Refinement of the Stetler/Marram model for application of research findings to practice. *Nursing Outlook 42:15-25.*
6. Joint Committee on Nursing Research and Studies. (1952). Research in nursing —philosophy and plan of action. *American Journal of Nursing 52:601-603.*
7. Simmons, L.W. & Henderson, V. (1964). *Nursing Research: Survey and Assessment.* New York: Appleton-Century-Crofts.
8. Fox, D.J. (1966). *Fundamentals of Research in Nursing.* New York: Appleton-Century-Crofts.
9. Abdellah, F.G. & Levine, E. (1965). *Better Patient Care through Nursing Research.* New York: Macmillan.
10. Hurd, S.S. (1995). The National Institute of Nursing Research of the National Institutes of Health. *Nursing Outlook 43:89-92.*
11. American Association of Colleges of Nursing website: www.aacn.nche.edu
12. Jacox, A.K. & Norris, C.M. (Eds.) (1977). *Organizing for Independent Nursing Practice.* New York: Appleton-Century-Crofts. pp. 205-206.
13. O'Toole, A.W. (1979). The expanded role: Issues and opportunities for nursing. In: *Power Nursing's Challenge for Change.* Papers Presented at the 51st Convention, Honolulu, Hawaii, June 9-14. Kansas City, MO: American Nurses' Association. p. 60.
14. Barnard, K.E. (1980). Knowledge for practice: Directions for the future. *Nursing Research 29:208-212.*
15. Wilson, H.S. (1992). Identifying problems for clinical research to create a nursing tapestry. *Image 91(3):64-65.*
16. Johnson, B.K. (1991). How to ask research questions in clinical practice. *American Journal of Nursing 91(3):64-65.*
17. Ford, L.C. (1979). A nurse for all settings: The nurse practitioner. *Nursing Outlook 27:520-521.*
18. Harris, M.R. & Warren, J.J. (1995). Patient outcomes: Assessment issues for the CNS. *Clinical Nurse Specialist 9:82-86.*
19. Askin, D.F., Bennett, K. & Shapiro, C. (1994). The clinical nurse specialist and the research process. *Journal of Obstetric, Gynecologic, and Neonatal Nursing 23:336-340.*
20. Cronenwett, L.R. (1986). The research role of the clinical nurse specialist. *Journal of Nursing Administration 16(4):10-11.*
21. Brodish, M.S., Chamings, P.A. & Tranbarger, R.E. (1987). Fostering a research focus for the clinical nurse specialist. *Clinical Nurse Specialist 1(3):99-104.*
22. Brown, S.A. & Grimes, D.E. (1993). *Nurse Practitioners and Certified Nurse-midwives. A meta-analysis of Studies on Nurses in Primary Care Roles.* Washington, DC: American Nurses Publishing.
23. Martin, J.P. (1990). Implementing the research role of the clinical nurse specialist—one institution's approach. *Clinical Nurse Specialist 4(3):137-140.*
24. Stanford, D. (1989). Nurse practitioner research: Issues in practice and theory.

The Nurse Practitioner 12(1):64-65, 68, 72, 74-75.

25. Denyes, M.J., O'Connor, N.A., Oakley, D. & Ferguson, S. (1989). Integrating nursing theory, practice, and research through collaborative research. *Journal of Advanced Nursing 14:141-145.*

26. Notter, L.E. (1975). The case for nursing research. *Nursing Outlook 23:760-763.*

27. Taylor, R., Crabtree, M.K., Renwanz-Boye, A., Perry, B. & Thrallkill, A. (1990). A collaborative approach to nursing research: Part I: The process. *Journal of the American Academy of Nurse Practitioners 2(4):140-145.*

28. Crabtree, M.K., Renwanz-Boyle, A., Perry, B., Taylor, R. & Thrallkill, A. (1990). A collaborative approach to nursing research: Part II: The findings. *Journal of the American Academy of Nurse Practitioners 2(4):146-152.*

28a Johnson, J.E. (1979). Translating research to practice. In: *Power: Nursing's Challenge for Change.* Papers Presented at the 51st convention, Honolulu, Hawaii, June 9-14, 1978. Kansas City, MO: American Nurses' Association, p. 125.

29. Miller, J.R. & Messenger, S.R. (1978). Obstacles to applying nursing research findings. *American Journal of Nursing 78:632-634.*

30. King, D., Barnard, K.E. & Hoehn, R. (1981). Disseminating the results of nursing research. *Nursing Research 29:164-169.*

31. Hickey, M. (1990). The role of the clinical nurse specialist in the research utilization process. *Clinical Nurse Specialist 4(2):93-96.*

32. Stetler, C.B. & Dimaggio, G. (1991). Research utilization among clinical nurse specialists. *Clinical Nurse Specialist 5(3):151-155.*

33. Douglas, S., Hill, M.N. & Cameron, E.M. (1989). Clinical nurse specialist: A facilitator for clinical research. *Clinical Nurse Specialist 3(1):12-15.*

34. Raudonis, B.M.. & Griffith, H. (1991). Model for integrating health services research and health care policy formulation. *Nursing and Health Care 12:32-36.*

35. Stetler, C.B. & Marram, G. (1976). Evaluating research findings for applicability in practice. *Nursing Outlook 24:559-563.*

36. Styles, M.M. (1978). Why publish? *Image 10:28-32.*

37. Diers, D. (1980). Why write? Why publish? *Image 13:3-8.*

38. Swanson, E.A., McCloskey, J.C. & Bodensteiner A. (1991). Publishing opportunities for nurses: A comparison of 92 U.S. journals. *Image 23(1):33-38.*

39. Grace, H.K. (1980). For the refereed journal. *Nursing Outlook 28:423.*

40. Lewis, E.P. (1980). A peerless publication. Editorial. *Nursing Outlook 28:225-226.*

41. Huber, G.L. (1994). Clinical nurse specialist and staff nurse colleagues integrating nursing research with clinical practice. *Clinical Nurse Specialist 8:118-121.*

42. Lewis, E.P. (1982). For the nurse writer's bookshelf. *American Journal of Nursing 82(7):1116-1118.*

43. Hodgman, E.C. (1980). On writing and writing workshops. *Nursing Outlook 28:366-371.*

44. Johnson, S.H. (1989). Finding time to write within a busy CNS schedule. *Momentum 7(2):1; 3-4.*
45. Swanson, E. & McCloskey, J.C. (1982). The manuscript review process of nursing journals. *Image 14:72-76.*
46. Gay, J.T. & Edgil, A.E. (1989). When your manuscript is rejected. *Nursing and Health Care 10(8):459-461.*
47. Hawkins, J.W. & Matteson, P.S. (1993). Using statistical software and a personal computer for on-site direct data entry and analysis. *Journal of the American Academy of Nurse Practitioners 5(3):125-129.*
48. Wu, Y.B., Crosby, F., Ventura, M. & Finnick, M. (1995). In a changing world: Database to keep the pace. *Clinical Nurse Specialist 8:104-108.*
49. Silva, M. (1995). *Ethical Guidelines in the Conduct, Dissemination and Implementation of Nursing Research.* Washington, DC: American Nurses Publishing.
50. Loos, F.D., Shortridge, H.A., Adaskin, E.J., & Rock, B.L. (1994). When industry courts your clinical skills, should you collaborate? *Clinical Nurse Specialist 8:85-89.*
51. Wells, N. & Baggs, J. Survey of practicing nurses' research interests and activities. *Clinical Nurse Specialist 8:145-151.*
52. Krywanio, M.L. (1994). Integrating research into private practice through consultation. *Nurse Practitioner 19(2):47-50.*
53. Turner, B.S. & Weiss, M. (1994). How to make research happen: Working with staff. *Journal of Obstetric, Gynecologic, and Neonatal Nursing 23:345-349.*
54. American Association of Critical-Care Nurses Thunder Project® Task Force. (1995). Nurses' perceptions of involvement in Thunder Project®. *Clinical Nurse Specialist 9:88-91.*
55. Gennaro, S. (1994). Research utilization: An overview. *Journal of Obstetric, Gynecologic, and Neonatal Nursing 23:313-319.*
56. Bonnel, W.B. (1994). Sharing your research project: A continuing education approach. *Clinical Nurse Specialist 8:92-96.*
57. Buppert, C.K. (1995). Justifying nurse practitioner existence: Hard facts to hard figures. *Nurse Practitioner 20(8):43-44, 46-48.*
58. Thibodeau, J. & MacRae, J. (1997). Breast cancer survival: A phenomenological inquiry. *Advanced in Nursing Science 19:65-74.*
59. Gaus, C.R. & Fraser, I. (1996). Shifting paradigms and the role of research. *Health Affairs 15(2):235-242.*
60. Hamric, A.B. (1998). Using research to influence the regulatory process. *Advanced Practice Nursing Quarterly 4(3):44-50.*
61. Doty, R.E. (1997). Advancing the role of clinical nurse specialist in rural family health research. *Clinical Nurse Specialist 11(1):2-5.*
62. Raybuck, J.A. (1997). The clinical nurse specialist as research coordinator in clinical drug trials. *Clinical Nurse Specialist 11(1):15-19.*
63. Grey, M. & Walker, P:.H. (1998). Practice-based research networks for nursing. *Nursing Outlook 46(3):125-129.*
64. Oates, K. (1997). Models of planned change and research utilization applied

to product evaluation. *Clinical Nurse Specialist 11(6):270-273.*
65. Carroll, D.L., Greenwood, R., Lynch, K.E., et al. (1997). Barriers and facilitators to the utilization of nursing research. *Clinical Nurse Specialist 11(5):207-212.*
66. Goldberg, N.J.(1998). An advanced practice nurse-nurse researcher collaborative model. *Clinical Nurse Specialist 12(6):251-255.*
67. Imle, M.A. (1998). Defining a place for clinical nursing research in the spheres of CNS influence. *Clinical Nurse Specialist 12(6):230-231.*
68. Morin, K.H., Bucher, L., Plowfield, L., et al. (1999). Using research to establish protocols for practice: A statewide study of acute care agencies. *Clinical Nurse Specialist 13(2):77-84.*

BIBLIOGRAPHY

Annual Review of Nursing Research. (1983-1999). New York: Springer

Bernstein, J., Bernstein, A.B., & Shannon, T. (Eds). Building bridges between the HMO and health services research committees. *Medical Care Research and Review 53(suppl.):S5-S145.*

Blancett, S.S. (1991). The ethics of writing and publishing. *Journal of Nursing Administration 21:31-36.*

Blancett, S.S. (1991). Who is entitled to authorship? *Nurse Educator 16(5):3.*

Blancett, S.S. (1988). The process and politics of writing for publication. *Clinical Nurse Specialist 2(3):113-117.*

Blancett, S.S., Flanagin, A. & Young, R.K. (1995). Duplicate publication in the nursing literature. *Image 27(1):51-56.*

Boykoff, S.L. (1989). Coauthorship: Collaboration without conflict. *American Journal of Nursing 89(9):1164.*

Bradigan, P.S., Powell, C.A., & Van Brimmer, B. (Eds). (1998). *Writer's Guide to Nursing and Allied Health Journals.* Washington, DC: American Nurses Publishing.

Brooten, D.E. (1986). Who's on first? *Nursing Research 35:259.*

Burns, N. & Grove, S.K. (1999). *Understanding Nursing Research.* (2nd ed.) Philadelphia: Saunders.

Cameron, J.W. & Stiles, R.A. (1998). A framework for analyzing and improving nurse practitioners' access to research literature. *Clinical Excellence for Nurse Practitioners 2:115-120.*

Camillieri, R. (1987). Six ways to write right. *Image 19:210-212.*

Collins, B.A. (1994). Creating and presenting an effective poster. *AWHONN Voice 2(3):14-15.*

Edgil, A.E. & Gay, J.T. (1983). Nurses can write for publication. *Journal of Obstetric, Gynecologic and Neonatal Nursing 12:231-235.*

Fawdry, M.K. & Temple, A. (1989). Even in research, the medium is the message ...audiovisual materials for research presentations. *Western Journal of Nursing Research 11(4):502-505.*

Fitzpatrick, J.J. (1990). The power of the written word. *Applied Nursing Research:*

3(1)1.

Fitzpatrick, J.J. (1988). The joys and triumphs of clinical nursing research. *Applied Nursing Research 1(3):107-108.*

Fondiller, S.H. (1992). *The Writer's Workbook.* New York: National League for Nursing.

Fondiller, S.H. & Nerone, B.J. (1993). *Health Professionals Stylebook: Putting Your Language to Work.* New York: National League for Nursing.

Freund, C.M. & Fox, J.A. (1999). Research in support of nurse practitioners. In M.D. Mezey & D.O. McGivern (eds.), *Nurses, Nurse Practitioners* (3rd ed., pp. 32-71). New York: Springer.

Gay, J.T., Lavender, M.G., & McCard, N. (1987). Nurse educator views of assignment of authorship credits. *Image 19:134-137.*

Hanson, S.M.H. (1988). Collaborative research and authorship credit: Beginning guidelines. *Nursing Research 37:49-52.*

Harding, S. (ed.) (1987). *Feminism & Methodology.* Indianapolis, IN: Indiana University Press.

Holmstrom, L.L. & Burgess, A.W. (1982). Low-cost research: A project on a shoestring. *Nursing Research 31:123-125.*

Jackle, M. (1989). Presenting research to nurses in clinical practice. *Applied Nursing Research 2(4):191-193.*

Jimenez, S.L.M. (1991). Consumer journalism: A unique nursing opportunity. *Image: 23(1):47-49.*

Kelly, J.A. & Gay, J.T. (1990). Grantsmanship: The process/the art. *Nursing and Health Care 11(7):346-352.*

Kemp, C. (1991). A practical approach to writing successful grant proposals. The Nurse Practitioner 16(11):51; 55-56.

Kilby, S.A., Rupp, L.F., Fishel, C.C. & Brecht, M. (1991). Changes in nursing's periodical literature: 1975-1985. *Nursing Outlook 39(2):82-86.*

King, D., Barnard, K.E. & Hoehn, R. (1981). Disseminating the results of nursing research. *Nursing Research 29:164-169.*

Massachusetts Nurses Association. (1991). *Getting the Word Out: A Guide to Sharing Research Results.* Canton, MA:MNA

McConnell, E.A. (1995). Nursing publications outside the United States. *Image 27:225-29.*

Morse, J.M. (Ed.) (1991). *Qualitative Nursing Research* (rev. ed.) Newbury Park, CA: Sage.

Morse, J.M. (Ed.) (1994). *Critical Issues in Qualitative Research Methods.* Thoussand Oaks, CA: Sage.

Parse, R.R. (1990). Making more out of less...Publishing the same manuscript in more than one journal.0 *Nursing Science Quarterly 2(4):155.*

Perry, S.E. (1989). Misuse of common words. *Research in Nursing and Health 12(3):iii-iv.*

Polit, D. & Hungler, B. (1998). *Nursing Research: Principles and Methods.* (6th ed.) Philadelphia: Lippincott.

Publication Manual of the American Psychological Association. 4th. ed. (1994).

Washington, DC: American Psychological Association.

Reinharz, S. (1992). *Feminist Methods in Social Research.* New York: Oxford University Press.

Ryan, N.M. (1989). Developing and presenting a research poster. *Applied Nursing Research 2(1):58-64.*

Silva, M. (1995). *Ethical Guidelines in the Conduct, Dissemination, and Implementation of Nursing Research.* Washington, DC: American Nursing Publishing.

Sparks, S.M. (1999). Electronic publishing and nursing research. *Nursing Research 48(1):50-54.*

Tornquist, E.M., Funk, S.G. & Champagne, M.T. (1989). Writing research reports for clinical audiences. *Western Journal of Nursing Research 11(5):576-582.*

Yarbro, C.H. (1995). Duplicate publication: Guidelines for nurse authors and editors. *Image 27(1):57.*

ON-LINE RESOURCES

Website on nursing research: **http://www.windsor.igs.net/~nhodgins**

CINAHL index of nursing and allied health literature. Not free but accessible through libraries at no cost: **www.cinahl.com**

National Library of Medicine indexes: **www.ncbi.nlm.gov/PubMed**

National Library of Medicine Integrated Library System, Locatorplus: **www.nlm.nih.gov**

Assist NPs by use of electronic media: **www.npeducation.com**

Nursing Research Registry of the Virginia Henderson International Nursing Library: **www.stti.iupui.edu/rnr**

Instructions for authors for many health-related journals: **www.mco.edu:80/lib/instr/libinsta.html**

Funding sources for research: **www.rwif.org/main.html**

Grants for research funding: **nlm.nih/gove/ep/extramural/html**

Royal Windsor Society for Nursing Research: **www.windsor.igs.net/~nhodgins/list99/main/htm**

Health and Behavior Research, Center for the Advancement of Health: **www.cfah.org/FundingDirectory/intrafundingdirectory.htm**

4

The Advanced Practice Nurse
as Change Agent

Introduction

Advanced practice nurses have been called the mavericks and risk-takers of the profession. Certainly, they are often in prime positions to implement changes in health care delivery and respond creatively to the rapid changes and chaos that characterize health care today. They can also help to define for the public what nurses can offer to their patients and help to effect a change in the stereotyping of nurses (1). They can be instrumental in redefining priorities for the health care system by shifting the focus from illness to wellness and from medical care to health care (18). They can influence health care policy. Finally, they can help restructure the system of reimbursement for care so as to improve access to care for patients and recognize the expertise of all members of the health care team.

In order to bring about change, however, it is important to understand something about change strategies. Selection of the appropriate strategy can influence the outcome of the process and help to assure not only that change occurs, but also that it is lasting (if it is meant to be).

Initiating Change

Change comes about as the result of goal setting or identifying a problem (2). Some stimulus must be present for change to occur. Change may be planned or unplanned. Planned changes are designed to improve living, working, or recreational conditions in some way (3). In general, changes in health care delivery are aimed at improving the quality of care. For advanced practice nurses, delivery of optimum care for patients is central (4). Changes may also be directed at improving the satisfaction of those who give care or altering the setting in which care occurs. Thus, change may be directed at any one or all of three domains: structure (e.g., where care is delivered), process (e.g., how care is delivered and by whom), and outcome (e.g., quality of care, patient outcomes, and patient satisfaction with care).

Unplanned change is change that is not desired by those in power. The results may, therefore, be unpredictable and unintended. It should be mentioned, however, that unplanned change is not always negative and, in fact, may have some important benefits for those whom it affects (3). The unforeseen resignation of the nurse administrator of an ambulatory service may result in the hiring of a new person with exciting and revolutionary ideas with regard to nurses' roles in ambulatory care. A change from young families to older adults in a neighborhood will profoundly affect the kinds of health care services that are required. Short lengths of stay in hospitals provide opportunities for advanced practice nurses in community settings. The growth of managed care as a major force in health care and the development of care systems offer challenges and opportunities.

Initiation of planned change requires acknowledging 1) that there is a problem to which a solution may be found, and 2) that change is necessary. Those who would argue that nursing is a closed system which still clings to outmoded traditions and procedures should recall how Florence Nightingale used her gift of leadership to fight the existing health care system and used all the political power she could muster to bring about change (5).

At the same time that we have been digging in our heels and resisting change in nursing, we have also been part of the dramatic changes within our profession over the past 130 plus years. Nursing has witnessed profound changes in its structure, educational objectives, and practice since Nightingale initiated the transition to professional status. We have moved to learning-based education, the development of baccalaureate and graduate programs, research, theory bases for practice, and new roles and specialties. It is evident that nurses have been involved in change across the decades. Nonetheless, resistance to change still occurs (3, 4). It is incumbent upon the nurse who becomes a change agent to make a case for change and convince his or her peers that change will, in the long run, benefit both the patient and the profession.

Because health care agencies and institutions are often very complex, especially in this age of care systems and managed care, an organizational analysis can be useful prior to initiating change (26). Such an analysis not only helps to clarify needed changes, but also helps to identify the key players, the driving and restraining forces, and the change strategies that might be most effective.

Developing opportunities for advanced practice nurses to practice sometimes requires assessment of the climate for such practice in agencies, institutions, or care systems, or in a geographic region such as a rural area of a state or an entire state. Data are available to assist in this effort. The annual update of legislation for advanced practice is one source (11). Safriet's work provides information on the driving and restraining forces for two advanced practice roles—nurse-midwife and nurse practitioner (12, 31). Other research focuses on facilitators and barriers to practice for the clinical nurse specialist, nurse practitioner, nurse-midwife, and all advanced practice nurses (13, 14, 15, 16, 17).

Nurses in Advanced Practice as Change Agents

Mauksch and Miller have identified three characteristics of change agents (3). The first of these is being a risk-taker. The very nature of the advanced practitioner's role implies that these nurses are willing to try new identities and take on new aspects of their prac-tice and increased accountability.

Changes in identity and function occur when a nurse acquires the knowledge and skills to practice the new role of nurse practitio-ner, nurse-midwife, nurse anesthetist, or clinical specialist.

Assuming the role requires a commitment to practice that a basic program has usually not prepared one for. It may mean giving up stereotypic images of what a nurse is, does, and should be. Participating as a colleague on the health care delivery team may be a new experience. Every change agent must possess competence as a practitioner, skills in interpersonal relations, and a knowledge of nursing based on research findings and basic scientific information (3). As an organizational development consultant, an advanced practice nurse may be in a prime position to help initiate change (1, 4, 27).

Theories of Change and Change Strategies

Kurt Lewin, the source of classical change theory, viewed change as occurring in three steps: unfreezing, moving, and refreezing.

Unfreezing means getting people to think differently about a problem or a way of doing things. Some strategies to promote unfreezing might be to bring in a consultant, have a workshop, use previous research, and compile literature to support change. Another example of unfreezing might be to find out how many women in a prenatal clinic are the victims of abusive husbands/boyfriends by using a consultant to train the research team in using the Abuse Assessment Screen (AAS) (see bibliography, page 90), by designing and conducting workshops on abuse for the clinic's staff members, and by giving them literature that demonstrates the efficacy of the AAS in eliciting information about abuse.

Moving means trying something new, giving an idea a trial. Piloting a computerized patient record system in a faculty practice site and working out the bugs before implementing the system at other practice sites can help to introduce change in a way that involves staff members and recognizes and values their input (32).

Refreezing means solidifying the change so that it becomes universal practice. By adopting the Abuse Assessment Screen (AAS)

(33) as the tool to be used for screening all pregnant women in compliance with practice standards of the American College of Obstetricians and Gynecologists and AWHONN, it becomes a routine part of care.

Some of the driving forces supporting such a change as the one described above could be professional standards of care and fear of legal repercussions if the abuse of a woman goes undetected. If the children of a woman being abused are also victims, health care professionals are under legal obligations to report the abuse to the appropriate authorities.

On the other hand, health care providers may resist screening patients for domestic violence if they fear that they will uncover abuse and not know how to handle it or to whom they can refer the abused patients. Some providers resist the screening because they believe it will take too much time.

Kurt Lewin also emphasized the need to identify those forces that support change (driving forces) and those that mediate against it (restraining forces) (28). A number of other theorists who modified Lewin's theories are discussed in several articles on change and advanced practice nurses as change agents (1, 3, 4, 6, 7, 27, 29).

Chin and Benne in their classic volume on change describe three types of basic strategies: empirical-rational, normative-reeducative, and power-coercive (30). The rest of this chapter will examine these three categories for their application to the role of the advanced practice nurse as a change agent, and then some of the contemporary change theories generated out of their work and that of Lewin (25, 27, 28, 29, 34, 37).

Empirical-Rational Strategies
Empirical-rational strategies are based on the assumption that people are rational beings. The development of basic research in nursing and the dissemination of its results through education and the literature is one example of this kind of strategy. Nurses in programs preparing them for advanced practice roles may thus be

educated to practice in a particular model and incorporate the values of their preceptors.

Those selected for key positions in organizations affect the way nursing is practiced. A nursing director of a student health service who is strongly committed to implementing the role of nurse practitioner in primary care delivery can effect change in the way nurses are utilized. An elite corps of nurse practitioners may be utilized to demonstrate the role.

The Center for Advanced Practice at Columbia-Presbyterian Medical Center in New York City is an example of a paradigm shift in the role of the advanced practice nurse. Administrators at the hospital and the Dean of Columbia University School of Nursing created the center. To bring about this change, they undoubtedly employed empirical rational strategies, appealing to the bottom line as well as to the neighborhood's need for access to primary care, and used normative-reeducative strategies to teach patients and health care professionals about the ability of advanced practice nurses to deliver quality care (10).

Using those who are experts in implementing a nursing model for practice as consultants or staff can be one strategy to effect change from a disease-oriented medical approach to a health-oriented nursing model. Another strategy is to use experts in communication and semantics to assure that people in the organization communicate more effectively. Human relations training techniques can be used to improve both intra- and interdisciplinary staff communications. Life transitions theory is very helpful to nurses taking on the role of advanced practice nurse and to all nurses whose practice is changing in response to the chaos in health care delivery. It is useful, too, for registered nurses returning to the role of student (9).

Normative-Reeducative Strategies
These strategies are premised on the belief that humans are active beings and as such will seek to satisfy their needs and impulses (30). Humans are also social beings affected by the norms

of their culture as well as by internalized beliefs and values. To occur, then, change must involve the habits and values of the individuals and norms of the society (30).

Some of the strategies under this category involve use of change agents to involve the patient or system in working out changes. The change agent must be a consultant, researcher, friend, and/or therapist to the patient. In nursing, curriculum consultants may be utilized to effect change in an educational system. A clinical nurse specialist can be hired to demonstrate health care delivery for patients and providers. This person's success will be based partly on an ability to collaborate with patients and others in delivering care. For change to last, beliefs about advanced practitioners must be explored and value conflicts must be worked through. The dramatic changes in health care delivery challenge all nurses to create new models for care delivery and to use their expertise to meet the needs of patients and respond to the cost-consciousness of health care agencies and payment schemes. One example is an advanced practice role for an enterostomal therapy nurse who used normative-reeducative strategies to change the care of patients (4).

Psychotherapy is another example of a normative-reeducative strategy. Nurses are primary therapists for patients. There is also a movement toward more nurse involvement in primary care in mental health settings. An objective of therapy can be to help patients or families develop better problem-solving and coping capabilities (7).

Nurses in primary care often use strategies to help individuals, families, groups, or communities achieve growth and maximize the biophysical and psychosocial aspects of development. Strategies may be used to effect behavior modification, to achieve developmental tasks, and to reach or maintain a higher level of health. Partnerships between providers and communities can help both to achieve goals (19).

Staff development programs can be used to effect change in a system. Introducing and adopting problem-oriented records will involve normative-reeducative processes if nurses have been educated to use more traditional methods of recording. So will incorporating measures of patient outcomes (20, 21).

Power-Coercive Strategies

The use of power and coercion to bring about change is familiar to all of us. Nurses work in a system in which physicians have been treated as gatekeepers for that system. Traditional nurses' training stressed obedience, submission, and adherence to physicians' orders (23). Nurses have been the victims of power abuse rather than the users of power.

Using confrontation as one coercive strategy can be advantageous to nurses as a precursor to change (23). In some settings they may be grappling with role issues in relation to physicians. They may see themselves being used more as handmaidens than as colleagues in what is supposed to be a collaborative process of health care delivery. Planning is important if the strategy of confrontation is to be used positively. After using confrontation as a strategy to discuss issues, the outcomes should be evaluated (23).

Confrontation can be useful in effecting change when an advanced practice role is introduced. Nurses will have to use their expert power to implement the role; they may need to be confrontive in refusing to respond to physicians' expectations of subservience, such as demands to change the examining table paper, call in patients, or assist with procedures—unless these courtesies are mutual. For instance, one nurse manager used her coercive powers as a member of an executive committee responsible for an ambulatory clinic to enforce how her advanced practitioners were and were not to be utilized.

Confrontation can also be effective when used in appropriate situations. Faced with resistance from physicians over replacing regular beds with labor beds (LDR) that could be converted for delivery and recovery, a clinical nurse specialist asked a physician to lie flat on a labor bed. He got the message and the unit got the LDR beds (25).

In order to effect change, coercion is sometimes necessary. In implementing a patient education program, for example, it was necessary for one nurse manager to require all her advanced practitioners to participate. Left to volunteers, the program would have failed, as the same few individuals would have burned out quickly. Political activism through lobbying at local, state, and national levels is another example of the use of coercive strategies. The power of our vote will influence the actions of those who represent us. Nurses also hold political offices and serve in high offices in the National Institutes of Health, the Health Resources and Services Administration of the U.S. Public Health Service, and other departments of the federal government. There they can use the influence of their positions to chart the course of health care policy making (13).

A power elite can be created in nursing as in other professions to affect the course of nursing practice and to effect change. The officers of the National League for Nursing and the American Nurses Association might be viewed by some as a power elite, as might some of the specialty organizations in nursing and advanced practice groups (see Appendix G). Networking can be one way of connecting with the power elite of the profession (24).

Implementing Change

Goal/Problem Identification
The first step in implementing change is to delineate a goal clearly or identify the problem which has precipitated a need for change (25). What are the triggers for change? Economics? New discoveries? Consumer demand? Competition? Once we have diagnosed the requirement for change, we can determine what kind of change is needed (25). Do we desire to bring about a change in attitudes? An alteration in physicians' perceptions of the role of the advanced practitioner is one example of an attitudinal change we might want to achieve. The change may be technical; for example, the use of fetal monitors on all patients in active labor. Teaching patients self-examination of the breast is an informational change and, hopefully, a behavioral one as well. Adoption of the use of a computerized

record keeping system necessitates a procedural change. Reorganization of the physical layout of a clinical unit would constitute a structural or environmental change. Implementing care in a unit with labor, delivery, recovery, and postpartum rooms (LDRP) might be a role for a perinatal clinical nurse specialist and involve structural and procedural changes, and perhaps attitudinal and behavioral changes for staff members. Then it is time to consider designing a process or system to bring about change.

Contemporary Change Theory
Much of contemporary change theory comes from the education or management literature. McWhinney and colleagues (34) posited theory on modes of change. These authors describe analytical change as change based on data collected from the sensory realm which are then used to design solutions to problems. For example, interdisciplinary teams of health care and social services professionals analyzed data on homeless families and designed interventions to tackle the underlying causes of homelessness (35).

Assertive modes of change generally involve a charismatic leader or agent of authority. Florence Nightingale, indisputably a charismatic leader, changed both the delivery of care to soldiers in the Crimea and then the nature of nursing. Using influential modes, according to McWhinney and his colleagues, means imposing a truth on the group, focusing on issues of truth and fairness. Creating hospice units at a Department of Veterans Affairs medical center for persons with dementia of the Alzheimer's type happened because a few concerned and caring health care professionals used data about the disease's trajectory to convince other professionals that implementing a hospice philosophy of care was the most appropriate means of caring for patients and their families in an atmosphere of truth-telling and fairness.

In an *evaluative change mode,* change agents explore what matters to a group and find ways to distribute values fairly, using people skills for consensus building. An example would be the consensus building process that occurs when professional organizations update standards of practice and scope of practice statements. *The inventive mode of change* means translating ideas into material things. Artists, inventors, and entrepreneurs are the most obvious examples of agents for change. Often inventors and artists and entrepreneurs are not concerned with social values, but with ingenious and practical solutions. Nurse inventors have created new models for teaching breast self-examination to older women (36).

Finally, *emergent change agents* create ideas that reflect values, such as the activists who created the Habitat for Humanity program.

Recipients of Change

The recipients of change must be identified. Will the change affect staff, patients, the environment, the system as a whole, a subsystem, or some or all of these? How is the change to be introduced to those whom it will affect? Who are the stakeholders in the change? An acceptant intervention to get people to express their feelings and personalize the issues can be useful (25, pp. 18-19). Teambuilding sessions, termed catalytic interventions, can be helpful, too (25). McWhinney et al. provide a whole program for helping those to be affected by change examine their beliefs, values, and feelings and examine their responses to change (34).

Sources of Resistance and Propellers for Change

Identifying possible sources of resistance is helpful in selecting change strategies as well as in anticipating how the process will progress. This is known as force field analysis and is borrowed from physics. Will stasis need to be disturbed to effect change (upset the status quo)? (25). Is the climate conducive to change? (4) Will the change pose a real threat to anyone's job? Will the choice of change agent generate resistance? How best can the change be implemented so as to preserve the integrity of the system as a whole as well as the self-esteem, competence, and autonomy of those affected by the change? Where does the real power lie in the agency? How can the cooperation of this person or these persons be engaged? (34)

Strategies

Strategies to be used to implement the change must be appropriate not only for the type of change to be accomplished but also for the system. For example, coercive strategies may be acceptable when it has been decided to substitute one type of examination gloves for another; in this case, a simple memo to all those affected would suffice. When choosing a new nurse manager, however, similar tactics will probably elicit a strong response, and careful planning is necessary in selecting and planning the strategies to be used since the change is likely to affect others significantly. Those who will be affected by a significant change need to be informed about the process and the goals and educated for any new processes, procedures, or technology. Plans need to be made for any administrative adjustments that will occur as a result of the change or in order to support the project.

If possible, the change should be tested on a small scale before instituting it agency-wide. Introducing an advanced practice nurse into the pediatrics clinic may be followed by hiring advanced practitioners for geriatric and young adult services if the evaluations are positive. A new type of examination glove can be tried in one clinic before they are purchased for the entire outpatient service. Evaluating the pilot project will help to iron out any kinks before the change is adopted agency-wide (2). A psychiatric liaison nurse might begin work with a surgical unit and then, based on feedback, offer her/his services to medical, obstetrical, and other units. Change from a centralized to a shared governance model has a considerable effect on the role of clinical nurse specialists at a hospital (7).

Evaluating Change

Once a change has been effected, evaluation of the change and its effectiveness should occur. Beginning with a goal or objectives gives one criteria by which to evaluate the change. Has it accomplished the goal? If not, why? Are the means appropriate to the end? How have those affected responded to the change? (2). If advanced practitioners are hired for ambulatory service and, as a result, other staff resign, is the end worth the means?

Change should be assessed as to its effectiveness, efficiency, and satisfaction for all those involved. Longevity is an index of the effectiveness of change. Efficiency can be measured in time, energy, and dollars. Change is effective if it proves to be more acceptable, pleasing, and comfortable than the original structure, process, or outcome to all those whom it affects (2).

Last, it is important to report the change. Disseminating information about the change and evaluating the process and outcome can be helpful not only to those directly affected by the change but also to sponsors of the change (government, private foundation, agency administration), researchers and students, change agents in other settings, and colleagues in the profession (3). Internal and external communication about the change can be appropriate. Publication should be considered (3). One might say that until communication about a change has occurred, the process is not complete.

Summary

Advanced practice nursing roles underscore the potential for a strong contribution to, and strong leadership for, new models for delivering health care (18). From a grassroots effort, nurses created the Nurses' Network for a National Health Program dedicated to creating a universal health system that is single payer. There are now similar groups across the U.S. and increasingly they are multidisciplinary and supported by interested parties such as teachers' unions (38).

Change is inevitable as the present system is assaulted by technological advances, consumer demands for accountability and cost effectiveness, cost escalation, the role of managed care and creation of care systems, the women's movement, and changes within the profession affecting the images and roles of nurses. We have the power to be change agents, to affect the delivery of health care in our practices and to effect change for the system as a whole. "Planned change is part of today's nurses' leadership roles." It is, therefore, an integral part of the roles of the advanced practice nurses (1).

REFERENCES

1. O'Malley, J. & Cummings, S.H. (1995). Change . . . more change . . . and change again! *Advanced Practice Nursing Quarterly l(1):1-6.*
2. Stevens, B.J. (1977) Management of continuity and change in nursing. *Journal of Nursing Administration 7:26-31.*
3. Mauksch, I.G. & Miller, M.H. (1981) *Implementing Change in Nursing.* St. Louis: C.V. Mosby. p. 20.
4. Strunk, B.L. (1995). The clinical nurse specialist as change agent. *Clinical Nurse Specialist 99:128-132.*
5. Sparacino, P.S.A. (1994). Florence Nightingale: A CNS role model. *Clinical Nurse Specialist 8:64.*
6. Booth, R.Z. (1995). Leadership challenges for nurse practitioner faculty. *Nurse Practitioner 20(4):52-54, 56-58.*
7. Houston, S. & Green, S.. (1993). The CNS role: Evolution within a shared governance environment. *Clinical Nurse Specialist 7:87-90.*
8. Porter-O'Grady, T. (1994). Working with consultants on a redesign. *American Journal of Nursing 94(10):32-37.*
9. Barba, E. & Selder, F. (1995). Life transitions theory. *Nursing Leadership Forum 1(1):4-11.*
10. Hahn, M.S. (1995). The Center for Advanced Practice. *Advance for Nurse Practitioners 3(4):45-47.*
11. Pearson, L.J. (1999). Annual update of how each state stands on legislative issues affecting advanced nursing practice. *Nurse Practitioner 24(1), 16-18, 21-83.*
12. Safriet, B.J. (1992). Health care dollars and regulatory sense. *Yale Journal on Regulation 9:417-488.*
13. McFadden, E.A. & Miller, M.A. (1994). Clinical nurse specialist practice: Facilitators and barriers. *Clinical Nurse Specialist 8:27-33.*
14. Sercenski, E.S., Sansom, S., Bazell, C., Salmon, M.E. & Mullan, F. (1994). State practice environments and the supply of physician assistants, nurse practitioners, and certified nurse-midwives. *The New England Journal of Medicine 331:1266-1271.*
15. Pew Health Professions Commission. (1994). *Primary Care Workforce 2000.* San Francisco, University of California.
16. Lehrman, E. (1992). Findings of the 1990 annual American College of Nurse-Midwives membership survey. *Journal of Nurse-Midwifery 37(1):33-47.*4
17. Minarik, P.A. & Tyner, I. (1999). Update on clinical nurse specialist recognition and prescriptive authority. *Clinical Nurse Specialist 13(3):140-144.*
18. Bear, E.M. (1995). Advanced practice nurses. How did we get here anyway? *Advanced Practice Nursing Quarterly 1(1):10-14.*

19. Bushy, A. (1995). Harnessing the chaos in health care reform with provider-community partnerships. *Journal of Nursing Care Quality 9(3):10-19.*
20. Brown, S.A. & Grimes, D.E. (1993)). Nurse practitioners and certified nurse-midwives. A meta-analysis of studies on nurses in primary care roles. Washington, DC: American Nurses Publishing.
21. Buchanan, L.M. (1994). Therapeutic nursing intervention knowledge development and outcome measures for advanced practice. *Nursing & Health Care 14:190-195.*
22. Hawkins, J.W. & Higgins, L.P. (1993). *Nursing and the American Health Care Delivery System.* 3rd ed. New York: The Tiresias Press
23. Smoyak, S.A. (1974) The confrontation process. *American Journal of Nursing 74:1632-1635.*
24. Fain, J.A. & Viau, P. (1989). Networking: A strategy for strengthening the role of the clinical nurse specialist. *Clinical Nurse Specialist 3(1), 29-31.*
25. Maher, H. & Hatt, P. (1998). *Agents of Change.* Dublin: Oak Tree Press.
26. Reddecliff, M., Smith, E.L. & Ryan-Merritt, M. (1989). Organizational analysis: Tool for the clinical nurse specialist. *Clinical Nurse Specialist 3(3):133-136.*
27. Johnston, B. (1998). Managing change in health care redesign: A model to assist staff in promoting health change. *Nursing Economic$ 16(1):12-17.*
28. Lewin, K. (1958) Group decision and social change. In: E. Maccoby (Ed.) Readings in Social Psychology (3rd ed.). New York: Holt, Rinehart and Winston.
29. Sadler, P. (1995). *Managing Change.* London: Kogen Page.
30. Chin, R. & Benne, K.D. (1984) General strategies for effecting changes in human systems. In: W.G. Bennis, K.D. Benne & R. Chin (Eds.) *The Planning of Change* (4th ed.). Chicago: Holt, Rinehart and Winston.
31. Safriet, B.J. (1998). Still spending dollars, still searching for sense: Advanced practice nursing in an era of regulatory and economic turmoil. *Advanced Practice Nursing Quarterly 4(3):24-33.*
32. Wong, St.T., Bernick, L.A., Portillo, C., et al. (1999). Implementing a nurse information system in a nurse-managed primary care practice: A process in progress. *Clinical Excellence for Nurse Practitioners: The International Journal of NPACE 3(2):123-127.*
33. Tiffany, C.R. & Lutjens, L.R.J. (1998). *Planned Change Theories for Nursing.* Thousand Oaks, CA: Sage.
34. McWhinney, W., Webber, J.B., Smith, D.M. & Novokowskky, B.J. (1997). *Creating Paths of Change.* Thousand Oaks, CA: Sage.
35. Rog, D.J. & Gutman, M. (1997). The homeless families program. In S.L. Isaacs & J.R. Knickmnan (Eds.) *To Improve Health and Health Care 1997* (pp. 211-231). San Francisco: Jossey-Bass.
36. Wood, R. & Bruckner, F.M. (1997). Design and testing of geriatric breast model prototypes. *Clinical Excellence for Nurse Practitioners 1(3):177-184.*
37. French, W.L., Bell, C.H. & Zawacki, R.A. (1994). *Organization Development and Transformation.* Burr Ridge, IL: Irwin.
38. Nurses Network for a National Health Program (1999, Fall). *News of the Nurses Network for a National Health Program.* Richmond, VA: NNNHP.

BIBLIOGRAPHY

Abuse Assessment Screen. (1990). Developed by the Nursing Research Consortium on Violence and Abuse.

Kobokovich, L.J. (1997). Use of accelerating clinical improvement in reorganization of care: The Dartmouth-Hitchcock Medical Center experience. *Journal of Obstetric, Gynecologic, and Neonatal Nursing 26:334-341.*

Lamar, K. (1997). Implementing an immunization program in the neonatal intensive care unit. *Neonatal Network 16(3):41-44.*

Manion, J. (1995). Understanding the seven stages of change. *American Journal of Nursing 95(4):41-43.*

Oates, K. (1997). Models of planned change and research utilization applied to product evaluation. *Clinical Nurse Specialist 11(6):270-273.*

Vincenzei, A.E., White, K.R. & Begun, J.W. (1997). Chaos in nursing: Make it work for you. *American Journal of Nursing 98(1):26-31.*

ONLINE RESOURCE

Change: **www.collaborate.org**

5

Power and Nursing:
Need for a Paradigm of Empowerment

Introduction

The word "power" has many connotations. It commonly implies an ability to control others by virtue of one's authority or to sway or influence others towards one's own viewpoint. Nurses are the only authorities who can speak for the profession of nursing when issues of role delineation, nursing actions, or nursing outcomes are in question.

Power can also be viewed as a capability for action as in the ability to perform or produce. The advanced practice nurse gains access to this type of power through education and experience and through identifying resources which can be mobilized and brought to bear upon a particular situation to affect a desired outcome (1, 24).

The latent power inherent in the professional nursing role should be capitalized upon in order to help shape the future directions of the health system and nursing's role in it. The advanced practice nurse must learn to identify aspects of personal and professional power and to use this power to advantage by collaborating with nursing peers within the profession to further the public and political image of nursing as an autonomous entity (19).

The Roots of Powerlessness

The roots of powerlessness in the profession today can be partially traced to nurses' socialization in traditional female roles and the profession's relations with physicians and hospital administrators. Before professional autonomy can be achieved, nurses need to understand nursing's historical ties to the system that has held them powerless (2).

Nursing education has its genesis in hospitals under the domination of physicians. Fry maintains that, as a result, the nurse became fused to the hospital and physician in a dependency state (2). The fact that hospitals and physicians *needed* nurses and were dependent upon them to function was rarely capitalized on by nurses to develop a position of equality with the medical profession.

Florence Nightingale attributed *all* successful recoveries to the ministrations of the "proper" nurses. When Nightingale arrived at Scutari in 1855, the death rate for sick and wounded soldiers averaged an alarming 42%; under her management and the resultant sanitary improvements and nursing care, the death rate dropped to 2% in six months' time (3). In 1976, in Los Angeles and Bogota, Columbia, the death rate dropped 18% in the former city and 35% in the latter city when physicians in both areas went on strike (4). From these examples it would seem that Nightingale was more right than wrong as to who is dependent upon whom.

The slow erosion of nursing's power began in 1885 when Clara Weeks Shaw added qualifiers to nurses' independence. Shaw delineated the duties that nurses owed to physicians while stating that patients' recovery, in *some* instances, was more dependent on nursing than medical skill (5).

In the early nineteen hundreds, Bertha Harmer linked the entire profession of nursing to medicine rather than viewing nursing as a free-standing autonomous profession (6). As recently as the 1960s, some nursing leaders continued to espouse nursing's dependency. In the 1990s, under the duress of chaos in health care, some nursing leaders were capitulating again. As seamless systems emerge, nurses will probably be interdependent with other caregivers. We must take care, however, not to revisit dependency. Orlando conceptualized recipients of nursing care as being under medical care or supervision (7). In this instance, a nursing author explicitly stated that the client belonged to the physician. Is it any wonder then that medicine is viewed as possessing more power than nursing?

Since the time of Florence Nightingale, a long history of subservience to and dependency on physicians can be documented, a history which must now, at last, be left behind in order to further nursing's efforts in meeting its goals. Ashley accurately pinpointed the difficulties when she made the observation that the powerlessness of the profession today resulted from the ways in which nurses used, misused, and abused their power (or failed to use it at all) as well as from the system in which nursing developed (8). Fry states that, as a profession, nurses have to begin the process of divorcing themselves from those aspects of history which hold them back from independence and professional autonomy, thereby creating a proud legacy for the next generation of nurses (2).

Power as Influence

Within the profession of nursing there are many nurses who possess a great deal of latent power. Those in managerial positions, those who teach and those who provide direct patient care are all in positions in which they can exert a great deal of power. Why then is this latent power not tapped? Why do most nurses feel powerless? Viewing power in action and analyzing aspects which influence one's ability to identify and use power can assist advanced practice nurses to mobilize their own strengths.

Since Florence Nightingale, few if any nurses have risen to a position of public power within society. This is not to imply that the nursing profession has not had its influential leaders nor that power has not been exerted on societies by nurses. Rather, efforts by nurses,, when undertaken, have been exerted by collectives of individuals and not by loners. Nightingale, perhaps, stands alone, epitomizing the nurse leader waging a battle singlehandedly. Nightingale was responsible for significant organizational reforms within the army, the government, and the educational system. How many other nurses could boast of such broad and diverse achievements affecting complex organizations in society? "One of the world's most inspired and inspirational people, Florence Nightingale knew what she wanted to accomplish in her life and set out to do so, leaving a heritage rarely surpassed and seldom approximated in the history of women and of nations" (9).

One reason that nursing's power base has remained weak is that power tends to be associated with males, especially white males, and "men will go to extraordinary lengths to invent power structures. . . to deprive successful women of their autonomy" (10). Nursing's movement toward autonomy was thwarted when hospital administrators and physicians realized their dependence on nurses; this need was quickly expressed as a need to exert control over nurses (11). Florence Nightingale was astute enough to recognize and use to her advantage the need men have to exert power over women and the threat that a competent woman presents to them.

Nightingale capitalized on other persons' influential ties, involving them in her causes and convincing them that her causes were to their benefit. Her reforms were carried out by men she personally inspired (9). Perhaps it is also significant that, at the time, England had a queen rather than a king, a queen who personally espoused some of Nightingale's reform measures. Power is influence and Nightingale developed the art of influence to perfection.

Power as Ability

Professional ability is dependent upon education and experience. The persistent fusion of many nurses to the hospital organization has prevented many of them from seeing the need for or value of advanced education. Many of these nurses have been unwilling to augment their knowledge by a return to formal educational programs due to a sense of loyalty to the "parental" hospital system (2). Of even greater significance is the obvious lack of financial rewards once higher education credentials are attained. For men, education is usually directly correlated with income, social position, and occupational power. This is not necessarily so for women and, in particular, for nurses. McCarthy states that ". . . something is terribly wrong when experienced nurses, professionals who have worked full time for nearly twenty uninterrupted years on the staffs of hospitals and as university faculty members while putting themselves through graduate school are worth only forty cents an hour more than unlicensed graduates straight out of school. . . . In fact, in any other field, no one with those credentials would be working for an hourly wage" (12). Because of this, many excellent nurses with advanced education have fled from hospital settings into other fields of endeavor such as academe, only to find inequities there also. In university settings, women on faculties, including those in schools of nursing, despite having in their possession all of the necessary academic credentials, are paid lower salaries for equivalent rank and/or responsibilities than males (13, 14).

Hospitals have been the major focal point for professional nursing activities, employing 66% of all nurses in practice today (15). And, according to Lieb, ". . .it is in such institutions [as hospitals] that domination by male authority is most obvious" (11), a sentiment echoed by Muller and Cocotas (16).

Medical and hospital administration authorities have resisted and opposed baccalaureate nursing education since it was first proposed, for they understood how this would weaken their ability to maintain control of nurses (11). The lack of financial reimbursement for higher education credentials is only a manifestation of this resistance; the very fact that both groups continue to reap great financial profits while maintaining their secure power base at the expense of nurses should cause an American woman to feel some sense of outrage since it persists in a day touted as an age of equal opportunity.

Physicians were the first health care practitioners to achieve legislative recognition. The broad definition of medical practice makes it necessary for all other health professions to "carve out tasks or functions from this all-encompassing medical scope of practice in seeking legislative recognition of their own professional roles, no matter how traditional or long-standing their activities" (17).

Physicians have also used their political power to influence reimbursement policy and payment systems. For example, the federal Medicare payment system uses the Current Procedural Terminology (CPT) classification of payment codes, developed exclusively by the American Medical Association (AMA) to determine economic value for services rendered. Until very recently, the CPT committees were comprised solely of physicians. In response to strong efforts by the American Nurses Association (ANA), two advanced practice nurses were added to the committees (18). Although this is progress, nurses are still vastly under-represented on these vital committees.

Nightingale advocated ongoing education as a lifetime endeavor, stating that "no system can endure that does not march," and "to stand still is to have gone back" (3, p. 169).

> "Nightingale was an accomplished linguist, informed in the arts, mathematics and statistics, well read in philosophy and history, and perceptive about politics, economics, and government. She exercised her eager and keen intelligence constantly as she furthered her inquiry into her own varied interests, which included religion, philosophy, land-use systems, liberty, freedom, social conditions and institutions" (9)

In the creation of Nightingale's school for nurses, she founded a one-year program which would prepare nurses for health maintenance, prevention of disease, detection of illness, and care of the sick (3). But even a Nightingale had episodes of intellectual darkness, as when she simultaneously endorsed university education for women in general while she opposed the same educational preparation for nurses; perhaps she failed to correlate her superior accomplishments with her own excellent educational preparation (9).

This time of chaos and downsizing of hospitals is a great opportunity for nurses to uncouple their hospital jobs from their nursing careers and divest themselves of the "parental" hospital system. Perhaps only at the beginning of the twentieth century was there as great an opportunity for nurses to develop new and innovative models of community-based care—then, because there were few hospital jobs for graduates and now, at the beginning of the twenty-first century, for the same reason.

Power as Strength

Strength derives from a strong self-concept. A strong self-concept can be linked to a high level of motivation and success in one's career. Homer found that women demonstrate a need to avoid success and that, in particular, this avoidance behavior is aroused in women for whom success is a real possibility. The most competent women "when faced with a conflict between their feminine image and expressing their competencies or developing their abilities and interests, adjust their behaviors to their internalized sex-role stereotypes" (20). Sex-role stereotypes deliver messages which say that women have difficulty making decisions and are unable to act as leaders (21). Such messages affect women's self-concept, planting seeds of doubt about their ability to use their strength and power. Recent work by Veeder (22) refutes stereotypes of women as poor decision makers.

One of the better strategies for countering the effects of sex-role stereotyping is to identify one's personal skills and abilities as well as one's weaknesses and shortcomings. Knowing when one has the expertise to address a problem and identifying when external resources might be needed can facilitate success (19). Power can never be achieved without taking risks. It is of vital importance to analyze whether success or failure is most probable. Repeated failures influence one's self-concept, but a repertoire of repeated successes strengthens one's confidence in taking future risks.

Florence Nightingale demonstrated an ability to know when she needed to use external resources to implement her ideas and reforms. Not only did she collaborate and consult with other influential persons to achieve her reforms, she also gathered statistics and facts to substantiate her opinions and recommendations. When she addressed an issue, she presented written material which was lucid and graphic so that her conclusions were unmistakable; she did not leave it to chance that her suggestions would be transmitted in printed official reports. Instead, she privately published these reports and disseminated them directly to the British people. She used the public press, sending letters to editors and publishing lively treatises on necessary reform (9). Florence Nightingale's self-concept, rooted in her educational background and an accurate assessment of her own abilities, was, without a doubt, intact and seldom threatened by public opinion, rumor, or sex-role stereotyping. In the new millennium, nurses must work together to capitalize on their strengths and gain public support for long overdue health care reform. There are over 2.5 million registered nurses in the United States, one of the largest groups of health care providers. Nurses are the frontline care givers, yet the recent Woodhull Study on Nursing and the Media found that nurses do not achieve media recognition for their contributions and do not capitalize on media opportunities to articulate their worth to consumers and policy makers (23). The nursing profession would do well to emulate Nightingale's effective use of the media to gain recognition and power.

External Resources
In order to obtain and utilize power, the nurse must gain access to a number of external resources to add to his or her own strengths. The creation of the journal *Revolution. The Journal of Nurse Empowerment,* in 1992, is a step in the right direction.

In 1971, a group of nursing leaders calling themselves Nurses for Political Action met to develop strategies for increasing nursing's sphere of influence. In 1973, this group became known as N-CAP (National Coalition for Action in Politics), becoming the political arm of the American Nurses Association. N-CAP and state political action committees have had an active role in influencing public policy. Notably, N-CAP has voiced opinions on the Equal Rights Amendment and national health insurance. Membership in a political action group is a way in which nurses can actively exert power and influence on our future health care delivery systems.

The National Organization of Women (NOW) has its own nursing chapter called Nurses Now. Membership in such an organization not only helps to expand the nurse's power base but also helps women band together for mutual achievements that transcend subgroup interests. Nurses at the state and national level of NOW are working to influence legislators on bills relating to third party reimbursement and prescription writing privileges for nurses in advanced practice roles. "Political activism on the local, state, and national level is another step toward empowerment" (25, p. 516). Founded in 1996, the Nurses Network for a National Health Program is a grassroots effort focused on creating a universal, not-for-profit, single payer national health insurance system. Working on the state level, nurses and other health care professionals are working for health care reform (26).

Political success, such as the override of the 1975 Presidential veto of the Nurse Training Act and ANA's campaign for health care reform, is evidence of the power nursing is capable of wielding when members combine their efforts. Political education, awareness of issues, and group membership can all help bury the image of nurses as powerless. Empowerment enables nurses to participate in actions and decision-making within a context that supports an equitable distribution of power. "Empowerment requires a commitment to connection between self and others, enabling individuals or groups to recognize their own strengths, resources and abilities to make changes in their personal and public lives" (24). It is a process of confirming one's self and nursing.

Summary

A selective analysis on some aspects of power has been presented along with an historical perspective on power in action as it was demonstrated by that powerful nurse, Florence Nightingale, one of the few British individuals who emerged from England's disaster in the Crimean War with an enhanced reputation (9).

A knowledge of history can help nurses decide for themselves which strengths of the profession should be capitalized upon and which limitations should be discarded.

Advanced practice nurses represent a small minority within the profession. To remain isolated from the profession at large can only bring powerlessness. Power can be strengthened by unifying and consolidating nursing factions so that numbers can become important and meaningful in influencing the outcome of issues which impact upon the profession (19). In the words of Brush and Capezuti,

"What [APNs] need. . . is to join ranks with their own professional organizations to gain and strengthen power for the changes ahead. Organization leads to empowerment and to autonomy . . . ." (19, p. 269). (See Appendix G.)

REFERENCES

1. Claus, K.E. & Bailey, J.T. (1977). *Power and Influence in Health Care.* St. Louis, MO: C.V. Mosby.
2. Fry, P.W. (1977). The need to differentiate. *American Journal of Nursing 77:1452-1454.*
3. Dolan, J. (1983). *Nursing in Society. A Historical Perspective,* 15th ed. Philadelphia: W.B. Saunders.
4. Wallace, I., Wallenchinsky, D. & Wallace, A. (1981). Doctors may be harmful. *The Hartford Courant Parade Magazine, Oct. 4, p.23.*
5. Shaw, C.S.W. (1885). *A Textbook of Nursing.* New York: D. Appleton and Company.
6. Harmer, B. (1922). *Textbook of the Principles and Practice of Nursing.* New York: The MacMillan Company.
7. Orlando, I.J. (1961). *The Dynamic Nurse-Patient Relationship.* New York: G.P. Putnam's Sons.
8. Ashley, J.A. (1973). About power in nursing. *Nursing Outlook 21:637-641.*
9. Palmer, I.S. (1977). Florence Nightingale: Reformer, reactionary, researcher. *Nursing Research 26:84-89.*
10. Korda, M. (1975). *Power: How to Get It. How to Use It.* New York: Ballentine Books. p. 255.
11. Lieb, R. (1978). Power, powerlessness and potential nurses' role within the health care delivery system. *Image 10:75-82.*
12. McCarthy, P.A. (1981). To halt the traffic in nurses. *Nursing Outlook 29:509.*
13. Astin, H. & Bayer, A. (1975). Sex discrimination in academe. In: M. Mednic, S. Tangri, & L. Hoffman (Eds.), *Women and Achievement.* New York: John Wiley & Sons. pp. 372-395.
14. Conway, M.E. (1978). The acquisition and use of power in academia: A dean's perspective. *Nursing Administration Quarterly 2:83-90.*
15. Aiken, L., Blendon, R.J. & Rogers, D. (1981). The shortage of hospital nurses: A new perspective. *American Journal of Nursing 81:1612-1618.*
16. Muller, H.J. & Cocotas, C. (1988). Women in power: New leadership in the health industry. *Health Care for Women International 9(2):63-82.*
17. Safriet, B.J. (1992). Health care dollars and regulatory sense: The role of advanced practice nursing. *Yale Journal of Regulation 9(2):417-488.*
18. Jacox, A. (1997). Determinants of who does what in health care. *Online Journal of Issues in Nursing. Dec. 20.*

http://www/nursingworld.org/ojin/tpc5/tpc5_1.htm

19. Brush, B.L. & Capezuti, E.A. (1979). Professional autonomy: Essential for nurse practitioner survival in the 21st century. *Journal of the American Academy of Nurse Practitioners 9(6):265-270.*

20. Horner, M.S. (1975). Toward an understanding of achievement-related conflicts in women. In: M. Mednick, S. Tangri, & L. Hoffman (Eds.), *Women and Achievement.* New York: John Wiley & Sons, pp. 206-220.

21. Broverman, I., Vogel, S. Broverman, D., Charkan, F. & Rosenkrantz, F. (1975). In: M. Mednick, S. Tangri, & L. Hoffman (Eds.), *Women and Achievement.* New York: John Wiley & Sons. pp. 32-47.

22. Veeder, N.W. (1992). Women's Decision-Making. *Common Themes . . . Irish Voices.* Westport, CT: Praeger.

23. *The Woodhull Study on Nursing and the Media. Health Care's Invisible Partner.* (1998). Indianapolis, IN: Center Nursing Press, Sigma Theta Tau International.

24. Mason, D.J., Backer, B.A.. & Georges, A. (1991). Toward a feminist model for the political empowerment of nurses. *Image 23:72-77.*

25. Sheer, B. (1996). Reaching collaboration through empowerment: A developmental process. *Journal of Obstetric, Gynecologic, and Neonatal Nursing 25(6):513-517.*

26. Nurses Network for a National Health Program. (1999, Fall) *News from the Nurses Network for a National Health Program.* Richmond, VA:NNNHP

BIBLIOGRAPHY

Ashley, J.A. (1980). Power in structured misogyny. Implications for the politics of care. *Advances in Nursing Science 2:3-22.*

Bookman, A. & Morgen, S. (Eds.) (1988). *Women and the Politics of Empower ment.* Philadelphia: Temple University Press.

Cotton, A.H. (1997). Power, knowledge, and the discourse of specialization in nursing. *Clinical Nurse Specialist 11:25-29.*

Dossey, B.M. (1998). Florence Nightingale. A 19th century mystic. *Journal of Holistic Nursing 16(2):111-167.*

Ernst, E.K.M. (1996)l Midwifery, birth centers, and health care reform. *Journal of Obstetric, Gynecologic, and Neonatal Nursing 25:433-439.*

Fitzgerald, S.M. & Wood, S.H. (1997). Advanced practice nursing: Back to the future. *Journal of Obstetric, Gynecologic and Neonatal Nursing 26:101-118.*

Gerchufsky, M. (1994). Enhancing the image of nurse practitioners. *Advance for Nurse Practitioners 11:25-26, 45.*

Godkin, J. & Godkin, L. (1997). APN barriers in Houston. *Nurse Practitioner 22(4): 248-249.*

Gordon, S. (1997). *Life Support: Three Nurses on the Front Lines.* Boston: Little

Brown.

Hennig, M. & Jordan, A. (1977). *The Managerial Woman*. New York: Pocket Books.

Keepnews, D. (1997). Is health care regulation really dead? *American Journal of Nursing 97(1):66-67*.

Korniewicz, D.M. & Palmer, M.H. (1997). The preferable future for nursing. *Nursing Outlook 45:108-113*.

Lynaugh, J.E. & Fagin, C.M. (1988). Nursing comes of age. *Image 20(4):184-189*.

Melosh, B. (1986). *The Physician's Hand*. Philadelphia: Temple University Press.

Messias, D.K.H., Regev, H., Im, E., et al. (1997). Expanding the visibility of women's work: Policy implications. *Nursing Outlook 45:258-264*.

Murphy, S.C. (1994). Don't be a doormat: Personal empowerment in nursing. *Revolution. The Journal of Empowerment 4(2):66-68*.

Rafael, A.R. (1998). Nurses who run with the wolves: The power and caring dialectic revisited. *Advances in Nursing Science 21(1): 29-42*.

Rambur, B. (1998). Ethics, economics and the erosion of physician authority: A leadership role for nurses. *Advances in Nursing Science 20(4):62-71*.

Roberts, S.J. (1998). Health promotion as empowerment: Suggestions for changing the balance of power. *Clinical Excellence for Nurse Practitioners 3:183-187*.

Roberts, S.J. (1996). Breaking the cycle of oppression: Lessons for nurse practitioners? *Journal of the American Academy of Nurse Practitioners 8(5):209-214*.

Roberts, S.J. & Chandler, G. (1996). Empowerment of graduate nursing students: A dialogue toward change. *Journal of Professional Nursing 21(4):233-239*.

Selanders, L.C. (1998). Florence Nightingale. The evolution and social impact of feminist values in nursing. *Journal of Holistic Nursing 16(2):227-246*.

Selanders, L.C. (1998). The power of environmental adaptation: Florence Nightingale's original theory for nursing practice. *Journal of Holistic Nursing 16(2): 247-266*.

Sohier, R. (1992). Feminism and nursing knowledge: The power of the weak. *Nursing Outlook 40:62-66; 93*.

Wear, D. (1997). Professional development of medical students: Problems and premises. *Academic Medicine 72(12):1056-1062*.

Willis, E. & Parish, K. (1997). Managing the doctor-nurse game. A nursing and social science analysis. *Contemporary Nurse 6(3-4):136-144*.

Wolf, K.A. (1997). Jo-Ann Ashley: Nursing's voice for empowerment. *Revolution 7(3):56*.

Zerwekh, J.V. (1992). The practice of empowerment and coercion by expert public health nurses. *Image 24:101-105*.

6

___

Effects of Sex-Role Stereotyping on Leadership in Nursing: Need for a Feminist Paradigm *‡

Introduction
In this chapter we will discuss the pervasive and persistent nature of sex discrimination which has affected the nursing profession's ability to influence issues relating to health care delivery. A major issue is the advanced practitioner's autonomy vis-a-vis a male-dominated medical profession. Knowledge about sex-role stereotyping and the effects it has on leadership in nursing can assist the practitioner and clinical specialist to develop strategies for gaining influence in health care settings.

Sex-Role Stereotyping: Women and Nursing
The vast majority of nurses are women (1). In 1975, research studies revealed that "existing stereotypic differences between men and women are approved of and even idealized by large segments of our society" (2). The findings were similar nearly 25 years later and the stereotypes continue with the new millennium (1, 33). Sex-role stereotypes not only affect the way people perceive the behavior of others as appropriate or inappropriate but they also influence whether they classify such behavior as healthy or unhealthy. Men disproportionately hold occupational roles that enhance gender inequality and foster a social dominance orientation (3).

___

* With Pauline F. Hebert, Ph.D.
‡ In this chapter the practitioner or clinical specialist is referred to as "she" because the chapter deals with women and sex-role stereotyping. There is no intent to disregard the male nurse.

Sex-role stereotypes are dangerous cultural social patterns not only because they limit opportunities but also because they affect achievement and motivation and ultimately affect the self-esteem of otherwise healthy and competent women. Proponents of the defeated ERA (Equal Rights Amendment) are still struggling to achieve a legislative mandate to guarantee equal opportunity for women, but it is doubtful whether a law alone can reverse the tide and put to rest the myths supporting the contention that women are biologically and intellectually inferior to men.

In nursing, women have played games with physicians, allowing themselves to assume and maintain positions of subservience which foster attitudes of medical paternalism in their professional relationships. Such behaviors may have been appropriate for survival in the past, but the issues which have to be addressed in the health care setting of the twenty-first century require a change in functional role and subsequent changes in interpersonal relationships.

Women continue to be perceived as less competent, less independent, less objective and less logical than men (2). One of the major difficulties today is the unavailability of an appropriate tool to fairly evaluate women. "Women are studied— and study themselves——in terms of masculine constructs" (4). These tools have been shown to incorporate masculine bias so that ". . . 'female' can only come out as 'not male'" (4). Broverman states that:

> Women are clearly put in a double bind by the fact that different standards exist for women than for adults. If women adopt the behaviors specified as desirable for adults, they risk censure for their failure to be appropriately feminine, but if they adopt the behaviors that are designated as feminine, they are necessarily deficient with respect to the general standards of adult behavior (5).

Virginia Cleland (6) classifies sex discrimination as nursing's most pervasive problem and states that nursing's autonomy is a false premise since the important decisions for nurses and nursing are not made by its members. The nursing profession and its members have assumed, more often than not, a reactive position, allowing more powerful groups the privileges of decision-making and offensive action. In a successful suit filed against a Connecticut hospital on the grounds of negligence by an employed nurse, a hospital regulation was subsequently adopted requiring a *physician* to double check medications prescribed prior to administration (7). In October 1977, although two nurse practitioners were functioning legally within the framework of the New Jersey state nurse practice act in an HMO setting, the Board of State Medical Examiners nevertheless filed charges against them, accusing each of practicing medicine without a license (8). Both of these examples portray the defensive positions nurses so often find themselves in.

For too long, physicians have assumed the right to dictate nursing's role. When something unfortunate happens, as in the Connecticut hospital situation described above, they quickly take action to keep nursing professionals under the thumb of medicine. What little autonomy has been demonstrated in nursing has been allowed by physicians as a means of meeting their own needs and goals. Although changes in state nurse practice acts continue to be promulgated to acknowledge independent functions for advanced practice nurses and all nurses, physicians continue to challenge these. Analyzing this situation, Edmonds (9) draws the conclusion that physicians perceive nurse practitioner and clinical specialist functions as behaviors which indirectly impinge upon their power. She compares patients to resources and nurse access to patients as threats to the medical ownership of patients.

It seems reasonable to argue that a still predominantly male medical profession is at odds with a predominantly female nursing profession for reasons which transcend professional interests and needs and are deeply rooted in sexual discrimination. Ashley even claims that this is more than it appears to be and represents, in addition, misogyny (10).

Women and Society
Depressed women outnumber men by two to one (11). In a study of women physicians and Ph.D.s, 51% of women physicians and 32% of women Ph.D.s were significantly depressed and related their depression to sex discrimination in their work setting (12). In another

study, female physicians had a suicide rate 6.56% higher than male physicians and four time higher than American women in the same age range (13). It seems evident that sex discrimination affects even the most highly educated and competent women in America, damaging their self-esteem and emotional and mental health.

Women and Other Women

That successful women encounter prejudice and discrimination from males is difficult enough. It is often true, however, that females tend to judge successful women just as harshly. There is no "old boy" network of women to latch onto for encouragement and support. LeRoux (34) discusses the way women are prejudiced against other women, undermining themselves and others by using censure whenever a woman violates a stereotype. Sohier (14) is concerned with how nurses can imbue each other with shared power and a community based on trust. The legacy of patriarchal rule is nurses' distrust of other nurses. "Revaluing" other nurses and becoming increasingly aware of the power inherent in our different perspectives can sustain change to a supporting, caring, trusting community and empower nurses to change the face of health care.

Women and Economics

According to statistics, nursing ranks highest in prestige among the predominantly female professions, but it falls far short of the most prestigious male group, namely, physicians (15). The undervaluation of all work performed by women can easily be proven by analyzing salaries paid to males and females for performing identical tasks. Levitin, Quinn, and Staines (16) found that a $4,372 mean difference existed between male and female workers; only $914 of the difference could be attributed to achievement factors while a $3,458 disparity existed for illegitimate or discriminatory reasons, leading them to conclude that most women were receiving far less income than they deserve.

Without a doubt, an individual's self-esteem is closely tied to the economic worth of her or his occupational knowledge and skills. An androcentric society which places women at an economic disadvantage and where high economic rewards are far more easily attained by males is perpetuating a work environment which furthers the advantage of one group at the cost of another group.

In 1945, nurses' salaries were one-third that of physicians'. Today, nurses' economic rewards average one-fifth that of physicians' despite the fact that nurses have assumed more complex functions and are more highly educated than in years past (17). Whereas the gap between physicians' and nurses' salaries has widened, the gap between professional nurses' salaries and those of auxiliary nursing personnel has narrowed to the extent that LPNs by 1981 made 76% of professional nurses' salaries (17). By 1992, LVNs in hospitals made 63% of what RNs made (18).

In 1979, nurses' salaries were equivalent to secretaries' and significantly less than those of social workers, physical therapists, occupational therapists, and pharmacists (17). Public awareness of the worth and need for nurses has had no significant effect on society's willingness to reward nurses financially for the vital functions they perform. This economic undervaluation remains a disturbing example of sex discrimination in the work setting, but a 1992 salary survey indicated significant gains: the mean salary for nurse practitioners in hospitals was $41,887 and for clinical nurse specialists, $43,593 (18). In Chapters Eight and Nine, guidelines are provided for assessing a practitioner's financial worth vis-a-vis the number of patients seen and the amount of income generated by the nurse in a particular practice setting. Although the nursing shortage in the 1980s led to higher entry-level salaries, the disparity in salary between experienced nurses and experts in other professions still exists. In the lean, mean 1990s, salaries fell and jobs disappeared.

The 1997 ANA House of Delegates reported that nurses throughout the United States have experienced economic insecurities resulting from salary cuts, shifting of full-time to part-time employ - ment and, in some cases, loss of positions to unlicensed personnel. The ANA Economic Security Council is attempting to resolve economic disparities within the Department of Veterans Affairs (DVA). Registered nurses are faced with salary restrictions not applied to other federal employees and are excluded from cost of living increases awarded by congress to other employees (19). At the turn of the new millennium, economic equity for women and nurses is still not a reality (20-26). The National Center on Women and Aging has initiated a new program on women's education for retirement (POWER). Research conducted by the center found that, in 1998, three of four working women still earn less than $25,000 and nine out of ten women earn less than $40,000. Half of all women work in jobs without pensions. Most revealing, women's earnings average 74 cents for every dollar earned by men, a staggering lifetime loss of $250,000 per female worker (27).

A survey of 1,792 advanced practice nurses attending Nurse Practitioner Associates for Continuing Education (NPACE) conferences in 1996 and 1997 found that the mean reported salary for full-time practice was $54,463, with a reported median of $54,000. This represents a 3.4% increase from the 1995 survey. While steady increases in salary are evident over the past three decades, the disparity between advanced practice nurses' and physicians' salaries still exists despite the fact that the educational preparation, skill set, and job complexity of nursing practice has greatly increased (28).

Implications of Sex-role Stereotyping on Nursing Leadership
The advanced practice nurse who attempts to exert leadership has many problems. An obvious one is the lack of available clinical nursing role models upon which to pattern a leadership style. In the past, educators, administrators, and researchers served as nursing leaders and spokespersons for the profession. This will not suffice in the future because changes in health care delivery systems will pivot around clinical issues which directly affect consumers of nursing care. Clinically oriented nurses must therefore learn to assume positions of prominence within the profession at large.

The advanced practitioner has been found to be different from her nursing peers in that she is more self-reliant, aggressive, and competitive (29). Nurse practitioners, clinical nurse specialists, nurse-midwives, and nurse anesthetists appear to be better armed to deal with issues of sexism as they attempt to gain more influence in the health care setting. While these nurses appear to possess the traits associated with leadership, their success will depend upon a variety of functions and roles which they must assume in addition to their clinical roles and everyday nursing functions. The battle for leadership must be waged on several fronts. At the client's bedside, the nurse must articulate who she is and what her functions are. She must demonstrate excellence in practice by considering all the needs of a patient—from preventing illness, through acuity and/or chronicity of illness, and into the realms of health restoration or a peaceful and dignified death. With physicians and other health care providers, she must be assertive in articulating her personal philosophy of nursing. She must break loose from medical paternalism and assume a more pro-tective and assertive stance as patient advocate by leaving behind loyalties to institution and physician. As institutions downsize and even close, this position is even more important. People need nurs-ing care, not institutions.

Within the profession at large, the advanced practitioner can make other nurses aware that advanced practice nurses are legiti-mate nurses, putting to rest the notion that they are nothing but "junior doctors." These nurses need to actively participate not only at the specialty council level but also within professional organiza-tions. Visibility as advanced practitioners who can demonstrate concern and interest in issues which affect the broad scope of nursing practice is also important. It is time for the profession to pull down the walls which separate its members into isolated special interest groups. In this, the advanced practice nurse can lead the way (30).

The advanced practice nurse must extend her knowledge by increasing her awareness of societal organizations within which nurses function. She can learn to identify where power resides in these organizations and how this power can be mobilized to further the aims of nursing. She can work to increase her consciousness regarding subtle aspects of sex discrimination in the work setting and, when it occurs, fight against it so nurses can achieve the success and financial rewards they deserve. Gary and Sigsby maintain that the significance of a feminist perspective needs to be reaffirmed and embraced if the health status of peoples of the world in the twenty-first century is to be improved through health care reform (31).

Summary

Advanced practice nurses represent a very small percentage of the approximately two million nurses in the United States. Leadership is a viable option for all nurses who possess advanced practice skills and a strong knowledge base in the fundamentals of leadership. "It is imperative that nurses recognize the value and legitimacy of their own voices. Political action by nurses requires bold actions based on visions that reflect both feminist views of the world and nursing's commitment to caring" (32).

REFERENCES

1. Allan, H., Canty-Diggins, K. & Gill, B. (1994). Challenging stereotypes. *Journal of Clinical Nursing 3(6):327-328.*
2. Broverman, I., Vogel, S., Broverman, D., Clarkson, F., & Rosenkrantz, P. (1975). Sex-role stereotypes: A current appraisal. In: M. Mednick, S. Tangri, & L. Hoffman (Eds.). *Women and Achievement.* New York:Wiley and Sons. p.38.
3. Pratto, F. & Stallworth, L.M. (1997). The gender gap in occupational role attainment: A social dominance approach. *Journal of Personality & Social Psychology 72(1):37-53.*
4. Carlson, R. (1975). Understanding women: Implications for personality theory and research. In: M. Mednick, S. Tangri, & L. Hoffman (Eds.), *Women and Achievement.* New York:Wiley and Sons. pp. 20-21.
5. Broverman, I., Vogel, S. Broverman, D., Clarkson, F. & Rosenkrantz, P., op cit., p. 45.
6. Cleland, V. (1971). Sex discrimination: Nursing's most pervasive problem. *American Journal of Nursing 71:1542-1547.*
7. Demensey, G. (1981). Suit over death of a child settled. *The Hartford Courant, Sept. 25, p. B1.*
8. Adler, J. (1979). Guest editorial: "You are charged with..." *Nurse Practitioner 4:6.*
9. Edmunds, M. (1981). Non-clinical problems: Concepts of power. *Nurse Practitioner 6:45-49.*
10. Ashley, J. (1980). Power in structured misogyny. Implications for the politics of care. *Advances in Nursing Science 2:3-22.*
11. Weissman, M. & Klerman, G. (1977). Sex differences and the epidemiology of depression. *Archives of General Psychiatry 34:98-111.*
12. Welner, A., Martin S., Wochnik, E., Davis, M., Fishman, R. & Clayton, P. (1979). Psychiatric disorders among professional women. *Archives of General Psychiatry 36:169-172.*

13. Pitts, F., Schuller, B., Rich, C. & Pitts, A. (1979). Suicide among U.S. women physicians. *American Journal of Psychiatry 136:694-696.*
14. Sohier, R. (1992). Feminism and nursing knowledge: The power of the weak. *Nursing Outlook 40:62-66; 93.*
15. Greenleaf, N. (1980). Sex-segregated occupations: Relevance for nursing. *Advances in Nursing Science 2:23-29.*
16. Levitin, T., Quinn, R., & Staines, G. (1975). Sex discrimination against the American working women. In: M. Mednick, S. Tangri, & L. Hoffman (Eds.). *Women and Achievement.* New York: Wiley and Sons. pp. 326-338.
17. Aiken, L., Blendon, R. & Rogers, D. (1981). The shortage of hospital nurses: A new perspective. *American Journal of Nursing 81:1612-1618.*
18. Brider, P. (1992). Salary gains slow as more RNs seek full-time benefits. *American Journal of Nursing 92:34-40.*
19. ANA House of Delegates (1997). Summary of Proceedings. on-line: http://www.nursing world.org/about/summary/
20. Avigne, G.P. & Guin, P. (1998). Moving from an hourly pay model to a professional salary model. *AORN 68(3):400-402, 405-408.*
21. Boughn, S. (1992). An immodest proposal: Pay equity for nursing faculty who do clinical teaching. *Journal of Nursing Education 31(5):215-220.*
22. Editorial (1998). A decent pay raise. *Nursing Times 94(38):3.*
23. Holmes-Rovner, M. & Alexander, E. (1994). Compensation equity between men and women in academic medicine: Methods and implications. *Academic Medicine 69(2):131-137.*
24. Roberts, J. (1998). Women's work is undervalued. And so is nursing. *Nursing Times 94(38):21.*
25. Sylvester, R. (1998). Better pay for nurses. *Nursing Times 94(37):24.*
26. Tiffany, C. & Lutjens, L.R. (1993). Pay inequity: It's still with us. *Journal of Professional Nursing 9(1):50-55.*
27. Estrin, R. (1999). Women's best interests. *The Hartford Courant, Feb. 2:F7.*
28. Pulcini, J., Vampola, D. & Fitzgerald, M. (1998). NPACE nurse practitioner characteristics, salary and benefits survey. *Clinical Excellence for Nurse Practitioners 2(5):300-306.*
29. Edmunds, M. (1980). Non-clinical problems: Gender and the nurse practitioner role. *Nurse Practitioner 5:42-43.*
30. Schutzenhofer, K.K. (1988). The problem of professional autonomy in nursing. *Health Care for Women International 9(2):93-l06.*
31. Gary, F. & Sigsby, M. (1998). Feminism: A perspective for the 21st century. *Issues in Mental Health Nursing 19(2):139-152.*
32. Mason, D.J., Backer, B.A. & Georges, A. (1991). Toward a feminist model for the empowerment of nurses. *Image 23:72-77.*
33. Peters, S. (1999). Hear me roar: How gender affects NP success. *Advance for Nurse Practitioners 7(5):58-60.*34.
34. LeRoux, R. (1976). Sex-role stereotyping and leadership. *Nursing Administration Quarterly 1:21-29.*

BIBLIOGRAPHY

Ashley, J. A. (1975). Nurses in American history: Nursing and early feminism. *American Journal of Nursing 75:1465-1467.*

Bullough, B. Barriers to the nurse practitioner movement: Problems of women in a women's field. *Nursing Digest 6:49-54.*

Bullough, B. & Bullough, V. (1978). Sex discrimination in health care. *Nursing Outlook 23:40-45.*

Bureau of Labor Statistics. (1998). United States Department of Labor. On-line: http://stats.bls.gov.blshome.htm

Clemons, B. (1971). Women's liberation and nursing. Historic interplay. *AORN Journal 13:71-78.*

Connors, D. (1980). Sickness unto death. Medicine as mythic, necrophilic and iatrogenic. *Advances in Nursing Science 2:39-51.*

du Toit, D. (1995). A sociological analysis of the extent and influence of professional socialization on the development of a nursing identity among nursing students. *Journal of Advanced Nursing 21(1):164-171.*

Elliott, E.A. (1990). The discourse of nursing: A case of silencing. *Nursing Health Care 11:539-543.*

Ferguson, K.E. (1984). *The Feminist Case Against Bureaucracy.* Philadelphia: Temple University Press.

Fisher, S.S. (1995). *Nursing Wounds. Nurse Practitioners, Doctors, Women Patients and the Negotiation of Meaning.* New Brunswick, NJ:Rutgers University Press.

Gordon, S. & Shindul-Rothschild, J. (1993, Dec. 7). Nurses have had it with sexism. *The Los Angeles Times, D7.*

Heide, W.S. (1985). *Feminism for the Health of It.* Buffalo,NY: Margaret-daughters.

Heide, W.S. (1973). Nursing and women's liberation: A parallel. *American Journal of Nursing 73:824-827.*

Helgesen, S. (1992). Feminism and nursing. *Revolution 2:50-57; 135.*

Leccese. C. (1998). Who's making what—and where: The Advance salary survey. *Advance for Nurse Practitioners 6(1):30-35.*

Lovell, M. (1981). Silent but perfect "partners": Medicine's use and abuse of women. *Advances in Nursing Science 3:25-40.*

Roland, C. (1977). The insidious bias of medical language. *Nursing Digest 5:51-55.*

United States Department of Labor. (1998). *Occupational Outlook Handbook.* (Bulletin 2500). Washington, D.C.

Vance, C. (1979). Women leaders. Modern day heroines or societal deviants. *Image 11:37-41.*

Wheeler, C.E. & Chinn, P.L. (1991). *Peace and Power: A Handbook of Feminist Process.* 3rd ed. New York: National League for Nursing.

Wheeler, L. (1994). How do older nurses perceive their clinical competence and the effects of age? *Journal of Continuing Education in Nursing 25(5):230-236.*

Williams, C. (1995). Hidden advantages for men in nursing. *Nursing Administrat ion Quarterly 19(2):63-70.*

7

Mentorship

Introduction

Although mentoring is an ancient concept, it is only recently that nursing leaders have actively explored the benefits of mentorship to the profession. Every practitioner or clinician needs to make an informed choice about whether to enter into a mentoring relationship and should understand what effects that decision may have on his or her career development. This chapter clarifies some of the misconceptions surrounding mentorship and explores its advantages and drawbacks. The developmental stages of a mentoring relationship, the desired characteristics of a mentor and a mentee, and alternatives to mentoring are also presented.

What Mentorship Is

The concept of the mentor has its origins in Greek mythology. Athena, goddess of wisdom, disguised herself as Mentor, a wise old nobleman, in order to act as the self-appointed guardian to Telemachus, the son of Ulysses, during Ulysses' 20-year absence from home during the Trojan wars. Mentor acted as protector, advisor, and guide to Telemachus. It is ironic to note that the first mentor was a woman whose role was to guide and facilitate the career development of a young man. Until the women's movement of the sixties, writers paid little attention to the role of women as mentors or mentees.

Levinson (1), in *The Seasons of a Man's Life*, expands upon the roles of protector, advisor, and guide, and identifies additional mentor sub-roles: teacher, sponsor, host, counselor, and exemplar. In the role of teacher, the mentor helps to develop the mentee's intellectual and career-related skills. As sponsor, the mentor uses his or her reputation and network of personal contacts to facilitate the mentee's entry into the work place in order to promote more rapid career advancement. As host and guide, the mentor introduces the mentee into the informal social network or "locker room" where many of the influential career decisions are made. Advice, guidance, moral support, and nurturance comprise the counselor sub-role. As exemplar, the mentor provides a standard of excellence which the mentee can aspire to or surpass.

A mentor, however, is not just a teacher or a sponsor or a role model. A mentor is a combination of all of the sub-roles which comprise a true mentorship: mentorship is greater than the sum of its parts. It is an intense, sustained, long-term relationship between a novice and a recognized expert in a given discipline (2). Mentorship does not happen by accident. It is the result of a conscious choice by both parties. The mentor is involved with the mentee in both a cognitive and an affective relationship of trust, preference, and mutuality (3). Mentorship is a nurturing support system essential to the novice's professional development and career success.

Many have said that a career without a mentor is doomed to failure: a mentor is necessary and essential to career success. May, Meleis, and Winstead-Fry (3) believe that "mentorship and sponsorship are essential for the scholarly development of nurses and for the integration of the scholarly role in the self." They go on to say that "aspirations to scholarliness are not innate but learned; such aspirations are developed in some novices and enhanced in others through mentorship and sponsorship."

There are many books and articles that advise young professionals to identify a mentor and to get one as soon as possible. A mentor is portrayed as the means to get to the top of the career ladder in the most direct manner. Sheehy (4) states that, virtually without exception, the successful women she has studied have been nurtured by a mentor. Henning and Jardim, in their popular bestseller, *The Managerial Woman* (5), concluded that career success depends upon a mentoring relationship with one's boss or superior. Kanter, in *Men and Women of the Corporation* (6), reinforced Sheehy and Henning's findings, observing that the sponsorship of high level, powerful "rabbis" or "godfathers" largely determines who gets ahead. It would seem then that in order to insure career success every nurse should find a powerful "godmother" or "godfather."

Benefits to the Mentor
To be sure, there can be definite advantages for both parties involved in a mentoring relationship. Erikson (7) states that the prime developmental task of the mid-career years is generativity versus stagnation. Mentorship is one way of countering mid-career obsolescence and boredom. There is a sense of personal satisfaction and pride gained from seeing a colleague one has nurtured gain success and career satisfaction. In Maslow's (8) terms, mentorship may be viewed as the ultimate self-actualization: feeling good enough about one's self and one's achievements to generously and selflessly help another reach his or her potential. The mentoring relationship may actually help the mentee surpass the accomplishments of the mentor and achieve greater fame and recognition.

On a more practical level, a mentor can gain more control over his or her work environment by spending time on those activities which require particular expertise and by delegating other tasks to the mentee who is learning the skills required in the early stages of career development. A mentor's reputation can also be enhanced by a "following" of mentees who serve as testimony to the mentor. This enhancement of the mentor's reputation can sometimes lead to lucrative offers to serve as a consultant, conduct workshops, or become part of other professional endeavors.

Benefits to the Mentee
Phillips-Jones (9), Kram (10), and Fowler (11), among others, have lauded the benefits of having a mentor because it can lead to:
- more rapid career advancement
- greater knowledge of the intricacies of a given system or organization

- ease of acceptance into the socio-political network
- higher publication rates
- publication in more prestigious journals
- more research funding
- choice committee assignments

Mentorship can also increase personal satisfaction and self-esteem by having an esteemed and respected colleague pay personal attention to a young, promising novice.

Disadvantages of the Mentoring Relationship

Before jumping on the mentoring bandwagon, let us look at the other side of the issue. In the clinical setting particularly, a potential mentor may have an actual or perceived work overload and may feel that a mentee would contribute to that overload rather than help redistribute time and energy in a more advantageous manner. If a mentor does not enter into the mentoring relationship willingly and with a positive attitude, then neither party will benefit from the mentorship arrangement in the long run.

Blotnick (12) tracked 3,000 mentor-protege pairs over a three-year period and found that two-thirds of the pairs ended up disenchanted with their relationships. Because the mentoring relationship is an intense one, it is subject to the same stressors and problems as a relationship between spouses. Just as tension in a marriage can lead to dissatisfaction and divorce, tension in a mentoring relationship can lead to an unhappy parting.

A mentoring relationship may be particularly at risk if the mentor and mentee pair are also boss and subordinate. Blotnick (12) found that in cases of conflict in these pairs, 40 percent of the mentors dismissed the mentee. The mentor got tired of the constant tension and removed its perceived source.

May, Meleis, and Winstead-Fry (3) identify other potential problems inherent in the mentoring relationship: dependence, exploitation, and lack of individuation. Because mentoring is a nurturing relationship, a mentor may become too "motherly" or overprotective with resultant dependency and passivity on the part of the mentee. The mentor may make the career climb too easy for the mentee. This may ultimately be detrimental to the mentee who never learns risk-taking, problem-solving, and conflict-resolution behaviors. Creativity and independence may be sacrificed for the safe tried-and-tested path. Maintenance of the status quo is not only detrimental to an individual's career, but to the nursing profession as well. Nursing is still struggling with issues of autonomy, assertiveness, and independence. A mentoring relationship between two female nurses can be at high risk for the dependence dilemma.

In addition to a balance between independence-dependence, a balance must exist between cooperation and competition in the mentorship. Over-competitiveness or extreme cooperation by either party can result in one person being overpowered and exploited by the other. An example of this situation is the well-known "Queen Bee" syndrome. The "Queen" cannot tolerate criticism, collaboration, conflicting ideas, or sharing the praise for joint endeavors, all of which are the primary behaviors desired in a good mentor (13). The mentee may develop into a drone whose role is to stroke the ego of the mentor to the detriment of establishing his or her own individual career identity. Mentors can nurture positive self-care behaviors and provide the mentee with guidance in juggling roles. Self-caretaking is particularly important for advanced practice nurses and for all members of helping professions.

Choice of Mentor

Awareness of the potential pitfalls of a mentoring relationship should not necessarily steer you away from one, but should instead help you make careful choices. The choice of a mentor is a crucial one that requires careful consideration and exploration before a formal arrangement is established. The mentor is a person with whom you will work closely for a number of years. For starters, you should enjoy this person's company and like spending time with him or her.

If possible, you should avoid having your direct supervisor as your mentor. Issues of subservience, on-the-job conflict, complaints of favoritism by other colleagues, and the possibility of being dismissed are mitigated if you are not working directly under your mentor. Also avoid choosing a close personal friend, but choose instead a respected, professional colleague with whom you do not have a social relationship. Although a mentoring relationship is a close one, it is a professional association and issues of friendship complicate it.

View the mentoring relationship as a long-term one, but also as a temporary one. It is not a life-long commitment. Establish a three-year contract with explicit goals and objectives to be mutually reviewed on an ongoing basis. If the relationship is not meeting desired goals, it needs to be altered or terminated before irremediable differences occur. Mentoring, or a given mentor, may be beneficial at one stage of your career but not at others. In order for mentoring to be successful, both parties must believe it is meeting agreed-upon objectives. This can only be ascertained by frank ongoing discussions. It goes without saying that your choice of mentor should be someone with whom you believe you can freely communicate.

A review of the mentoring research yields some additional tips which might be useful in the choice of a mentor. You must select a person in whom you have trust and confidence. This person must have the ability to motivate you to do your very best. The potential mentor must be respected in the area of your particular interest and have proven leadership ability. The mentor must have a great deal of confidence in his or her own abilities and must be happy with his or her own career success.

It is also recommended that, ideally, the mentor be 8 to 15 years older than you are. This age difference provides a one-half generational split and helps to avoid parenting or peer dilemmas. There is no general consensus as to whether a same-sex person makes a better mentor than a person of the opposite sex. It may be easier for a mentee to identify with a person of the same sex, but over-identification may then become an issue. Mixed pairs, on the other hand, may have to deal with sexual issues and patronage. The best advice is to choose the person, regardless of sex, who is most compatible with you and can best help you achieve your career goals. Finding a suitable mentor is only half of the equation. Are you a suitable mentee? You must be ready and willing to learn, dream, and invest yourself and your time in an intensive, goal-directed relationship. You need to view yourself as upwardly mobile and embarking on a long-term career path with specific goals. You also need to care for and nurture yourself and be willing to do so in the context of the mentoring relationship as well as in the rest of your personal and professional life. If this is you, go to it and seek a compatible mentor.

Stages of the Mentoring Relationship

Like any relationship, mentoring has developmental stages. These stages parallel career developmental tasks. Recognizing the stages of mentoring can help both parties plan appropriate activities and deal with potential crises inherent in each stage. The first of the mentoring relationship stages may be called the *invitational stage*. This is analogous to the honeymoon stage of social relationships or group behavior. Both parties display their best behaviors while carefully testing out their visions of the relationship.

The globally positive feelings of the relationship are soon replaced by fears about how the relationship will actually work out and by the realization that much hard work is involved. The pendulum swings from positive feelings to uneasy or negative ones. This stage has been referred to as the *questioning stage*. This is an opportune time to clarify initial impressions and solidify the parameters of the working relationship.

The questioning stage is followed by, hopefully, the longest phase of the relationship, the *informational stage* or *working stage*. However, if earlier conflicts are not resolved, the relationship will continually return to the questioning stage and energy will be expended in conflict rather than in output. The working stage is the time when the mentee actually "learns the ropes," discovers the political networks and power sources, and learns the game plan and how to master it. The mentee should be involved in concrete activities such as special projects, committee work, clinical practice, teaching, research, and publication under the guidance of the mentor.

As with all relationships, the final stage is *termination* (14). Termination always has both positive and negative feelings associated with it. A mentorship may terminate before the time of the predetermined contract if there is conflict, changing career interests, or circumstantial factors such as a move to another location. The relationship may also terminate because it is successful and has achieved the desired outcome. The mentee is ready to move on and assume the responsibilities of the next phase of career development. Termination should not just happen abruptly, but should be planned and discussed, as were the other phases. An unresolved termination detracts from career success in the next phases of the career ladder. Wheatley and Hirsch (15) give a detailed account of some of the emotional issues involved in the termination phase and offer concrete suggestions for dealing with these issues.

Alternatives to Mentoring

If mentoring is not for you, or a suitable mentor is not available, there are alternatives to explore. One avenue is having multiple mentors as opposed to an intensive relationship with a single mentor. This situation gives you the opportunity to seek and receive advice from several sources and avoids the potential pitfalls of an exclusive relationship.

Publications which give concrete, career-related information can serve as "paper mentors." Examples of paper mentors are given at the end of this chapter. Career interest subgroups of professional nursing organization can also provide some of the services a mentor offers, such as the guidance and advice of experts in the field.

Networks can also serves as mentors. Networks consist of persons who know about the system, have achieved some measure of career success, and meet on a formal or informal basis. Networks help new professionals establish valuable contacts and often serve as support groups. Networking may actually produce a sponsor or mentor or at least put you in contact with those in a position to recognize and reward good performance and make crucial recommendations (16).

As the paper age gives way to the computer era of electronic communications, consider networking via the Internet, World Wide Web, or one of the many user network services specifically geared towards nurses. Your computer can put you in touch instantly with a network of nurses around the world who can provide feedback, advice, and practical assistance.

Conclusion

Mentorship can play a vital role in the career development of the nurse practitioner or clinician if that individual makes careful, informed decisions and choices. A mentoring relationship requires forethought and planning. Mentorship offers an opportunity to both mentors and mentees to embark on a mutually satisfying contractual relationship with beneficial career rewards.

REFERENCES

1. Levinson, D.J. (1978). *The Seasons of a Man's Life.* New York: Knopf.
2. Schmidt, J.A. & Wolf, J.S. (1980). The master partnership: Discovery of professionalism. *National Association of Student Personnel Administrators Journal 17:45-51.*
3. May, K., Meleis, A. & Winstead-Fry, P. (1982). Mentorship for scholarship: Opportunities and dilemmas. *Nursing Outlook 30(1):22-28.*
4. Sheehy, G. (1976). The mentor connection and the secret link in the successful woman's life. *New York 8:33-39.*
5. Henning, M. & Jardim, A. (1977). *The Managerial Woman.* New York: Anchor Press/Doubleday.
6. Kanter, R.M. (1977). *Men and Women of the Corporation.* New York: Basic Books.
7. Erikson, E. (1963). *Childhood and Society.* New York: W.W. Norton.
8. Maslow, A.H. (1968). *Toward a Psychology of Being.* 2nd. ed. New York: Van Nostrand Reinhold.
9. Phillips-Jones, L. (1982). *Mentor and Proteges: How to Establish, Strengthen,*

and Get the Most from a Mentor/Protege Relationship. New York: Arbor House.

10. Kram, K. (1984). *Mentoring at Work: Developmental Relationships in Organizational Life.* New York: Scotts Foresman.

11. Fowler, D.L. (1986). Mentoring relationships and the perceived quality of the academic work environment. In: P. Farrant (Ed.), *Strategies and Attitudes. Women in Educational Administration.* Washington, DC:National Association for Women Deans, Administrators, and Counselors (NAWDAC), pp. 77-83.

12. Blotnick, S.R. (1984). With friends like these. *Savvy 10:45-52.*4

13. White, M.D. (1972). The importance of selected nursing activities. *Nursing Research 21:4-14.*

14. Keele, R.L. & DeLaMare-Schaefer, M. (1984). So what do you do now that you don't have a mentor? *Journal of National Association for Women Deans, Administrators, and Counselors, Spring:36-40.*

15. Wheatley, M. & Hirsch, M.S. (1984). Five ways to leave your mentor. *Ms. Magazine. Sept.:106-108.*

16. Barrax, J.D. (1986). A comparative profile of female and male university administrators. In: P. Farrant (Ed.), *Strategies and Attitudes. Women in Educational Administration.* Washington, DC: National   Association for Women Deans, Administrators, and Counselors, pp. 59-64.

PAPER MENTORS

Angelini, D. (1995). Mentoring in the career development of hospital staff nurses: Models and strategies. *Journal of Professional Nursing 11(2): 89-97.*

Annand, F. (1997). The mentor commitment. *Insight 22(2):41-34.*

Beck, L. (1989). Mentorships: Benefits and effects on career development. *Gifted Child Quarterly 33(1):23-28.*

Boyle, C. & James, S. (1990). Nurses as leaders: How are we doing? *Nursing Administration Quarterly 15:44-48.*

Brito, H. (1992). Nurses in action: An innovative approach to mentoring. *Journal of Nursing Administration 22:3-28.*

Byrne, M. & Kangas, S. (1996). Advice for beginning nurse researchers. *Image. Journal of Nursing Scholarship 28(2):165-167.*

Cameron-Jones, M. & O'Hara, P. (1996). Three decisions about nurse mentoring. *Journal of Nursing Management 4(4):225-230.*

Crim, B. & Hood, A. (1995). Learning partners: Preceptor, mentor, facilitator, learning. *Seminars in Perioperative Nursing 4(1):67-72.*

Cuesta, C.W. & Bloom, K.C. (1998). Mentoring and job satisfaction. Perceptions of certified nurse-midwifes. *Journal of Nurse Midwifery 43(2):111-116.*

Dirks, C.A. & Gouveneur, M. (1998). Learning leadership: Students' experiences of a midwifery mentoring practicum. *Journal of Nurse Midwifery 43(5): 375-380.*

Ecklund, M.M. (1998). The relationship of mentoring to job satisfaction of critical care nurses. *Journal of the New York Nurses Association 29(2): 13-15.*

Fields, W.L. (1991). Mentoring in nursing: A historical approach. *Nursing Outlook 39(6):257-261.*

Glass, N. & Walter, R. (1998). Exploring women's experiences: The critical relationship between nursing education, peer monitoring, and female friendship. *Contemporary Nurse 7(1):5-11.*

Haas, S.A. (1992). Coaching. Developing key players. *Journal of Nursing Administration 22:54-58.*

Hayes, E. (1998). Mentoring and self-efficacy for advanced nursing practice: A philosophical approach for nurse practitioner preceptors. *Journal of American Academy of Nurse Practitioners 10(2):53-57.*

Hayes, E.F. (1998). Mentoring and nurse practitioner student self-efficacy. *Western Jounal of Nursing Research 20(5):521-535.*

Kirk, E.k & Reichart, G. (1992). The mentoring relationship: What makes it work? *Imprint 39:20-22.*

Madison, J. (1994). The value of mentoring in nursing leadership: A descriptive study. *Nursing Forum 29(4):16-23.*

Madison, J., Watson, K. & Knight, B. (1994). Mentors and preceptors in the nursing profession. *Contemporary Nurse 3(3):121-126.*

Mateo, M.A. (1992). Publication skill development in nurses. *Journal of Nursing Administration 22:64-66.*

Miller, F.A. (1992). Leadership strategies for professional development. *Journal of the National Black Nurses Association 5:54-60.*

Norman, E.M. (1997). Boosting your career with a mentor. *Orthopedic Nursing: 16(4):13-16.*

Owens, B. & Herrick, C.A. (1998). A prearranged mentorship program: Can it work long distance? *Journal of Professional Nursing 14(2):78-84.*

Palletier, D. & Duffield, C. (1994). Is there enough mentoring in nursing? *Australian Journal of Advanced Nursing 11(4):6-11.*

Prestholdt, C. (1990). Modern mentoring: Strategies for developing contemporary nursing leadership. *Nursing Administration Quarterly 15:20-27.*

Pulcini, J. (1997). Succession planning: From leaders to mentors—an open letter to experienced nurse practitioner leaders. *Clinical Excellence for Nurse Practitioners 1:405-406.*

Schneller, S. & Hoeppnerr, M. (1994). Preceptor development: Use a staff development specialist. *Journal of Nursing and Staff Development 10(5):249-250.*

Stewart, B. & Kruger, E. (1996). An evolutionary concept analysis of mentoring in nursing. *Journal of Professional Nursing 12(5):311-321.*

Vance, C. & Olson, R. (eds.) (1998). *The Mentor Connection in Nursing.* New York: Springer Publishing Company.

ON-LINE RESOURCES

(See also Appendix G on nursing organizations with e-mail and website addresses; see also columns in every issue of *Clinical Excellence for Nurse Practitioners: The*

International Journal of NPACE, volumes 1-4, 1997-2000.)

Resources for NP students:
   http://nurseweb.ucsf.edu/wsww/arwwebpg/htm
NP Listserv: **www.son.washington.edu/npinfo/html**
NP nursing links (United Kingdom and United States):
   www.healthcentre.org.uk/np/links.htm
Nurse Practitioner Support Services (including national job search listings):
   www.nurse.net/np/index2.html
Nursing connection:
   http://home.earthlink.net/~mjsevero
Advanced Practice Nurse Survival Guide:
   www.utc.edu/~utcnurse/projects/GL/index.htm

8

Economics of the Roles

Introduction

At the new millennium, advanced practice nurses are faced with opportunities for developing unique economic models of health care delivery. With the health care system in chaos, managed care systems emerging as a model for health care delivery, the creation of care systems, and the challenges of population demographics for the year 2000 and beyond, this should, in Starck's words, "be *our* time —a golden opportunity for nursing to be a major player in a redesigned system" (12, p. 16E). In this chapter, we will discuss the economic aspects of the advanced practice nurse's role.

Being an Employee in an Advanced Practice Role

The majority of nurses in advanced practice are employees of physicians, clinics, hospitals, schools, community and rural health centers, public and private agencies and institutions, and industry. As such, they are in an employee-employer relationship and are salaried. The economic aspects of practice as an employee are much less complex than those of the independent practitioner but have gained considerably in their complexity under managed care and the so-called care systems. It is generally the employer's responsibility to provide office space, equipment, supplies, and other resources, while the nurse has to concern her/himself with salary, benefits, malpractice insurance, and the uniforms and equipment which she or he is required to supply. Some employers provide malpractice insurance coverage for their employees, but you may choose to carry your own as well. It is important to keep a record of expenditures that fall under the category of professional expenses in order to receive income tax deductions. With the revised tax laws, it is best to consult a tax expert. Some of these items are listed in Table 8.1.

Table 8.1. Items that May Qualify for Deductions as Professional Expenses

Uniforms, lab coats, special shoes, stockings
Examination and other equipment
Professional licensure, prescriptive authority, and certification fees and membership dues
Subscription costs for professional journals and newsletters
Malpractice insurance
Costs of continuing education courses, conferences, seminars
Travel to professional meetings, conferences, and travel to and from place of employment for business purposes (meetings, home visits) excluding travel between work and home
Typing, word processing, photocopying, secretarial costs and supplies for professional publication which you must pay for such as envelopes, paper, labels, tape, printer cartridges, floppy diskettes, reproduction of photographs, grapic art
Per diem costs for attendance at meetings, conferences, continuing education including food, local transportation, tips, and lodging
Professional gifts and entertaining
Books, calculated on a time depreciation basis
Purchase of a computer, word processor, camera, tape recorder, fax machine, answering machine, or other equipment used for business — calculated on a depreciation basis
Child care expenses associated with work
Postage
Professional phone calls; membership and user fees in a computer on-line information service
Tuition for credit courses
Travel for consultation or meetings with other providers or related to professional publication
Printing costs for business cards and resumes, stationery, rubber stamps, name pins
Disposables such as batteries or ear cones for otoscope, penlight
Home office expenses if you have a business on the side such as writer, counselor, or consultant for which you receive income

---

The nurse employed in a nonprofit rural or community health center, or in a voluntary nonprofit agency such as a visiting nurse service, may be more involved in the financial aspects of the agency than the employee of a hospital, other integrated health care system such as an HMO, or a for-profit health care industry because positions may be dependent upon soft monies or, in part, upon contributions or donations. Part of the job, then, may involve grant writing or public relations work to generate support for the ongoing operation of the service. Employees of agencies seeking rural health clinic status may have to participate in a community assessment in order to demonstrate why the application should be considered.

More and more, employers are looking at productivity for an index of the cost effectiveness of nurses' services. Such evaluations must consider more than the size of the caseload or number of patient visits (23, 70) and should include a multipractice factor analysis of cost effectiveness to provide data to support the need for positions and for nurses as members of the health care team. Unfortunately, this does not always happen.

Increasingly, advanced practice nurses are having to justify their existence in health care agencies and institutions. One mechanism for doing this is to generate fiscal reports on the contri-bution of the advanced practice nurse to the organization (30, 70). One radical and innovative approach is for nurse managers within managed care systems to consider advanced practice nurses as constituting a portfolio of assets with reports on their contributions to the organization; managing complex patients and their families/significant others; teaching, precepting, and coaching other staff members; engaging the health care team in dialogues about ethical decisions to be made about care; incorporating research findings into practice in order to improve the quality and outcomes of care; and so on. (72)

Another means of justifying advanced practice nurses from an economic perspective is to explore creative practice models that use their knowledge and skills to the fullest (74, 75). Case manager is one such role. At one institution, clinical nurse specialists act as trauma case managers for patients with high resource needs (67).

Advance practice nurses can be leaders in assisting health care agencies develop case management models to assure that resources are in place as patients move across settings, to avoid readmissions to tertiary care centers, and to plan for care most appropriate for patients' needs and the most cost-effective means for delivering care. Advanced practice nurses are superbly skilled in assessment and identification of resources, creating databases to facilitate a case management model (68, 69). Evaluation of the case management model from the perspectives of both providers and patients can help nurses modify this approach to care (71).

Integrative practice models are another approach to maximizing use of the skills and knowledge of the advanced practice nurse. By developing intradisciplinary models for care delivery, individuals can use their expertise to contribute to the goals of a unit or an entire agency. Advanced practice nurses with special expertise can be available across an agency under such models and advanced practice nurses with different preparation could explore new models for implementation of their roles (61, 63, 73).

Collaborative Practice

Setting up a group practice with one or more advanced practice nurses and/or other health care professionals involves the same steps one would follow as a solo practitioner except that you may elect to file the necessary legal documents to form a partnership.

Collaboration can be inter- or intradisciplinary. Nurses with different practice skills, knowledge bases, and educational preparation can establish collaborative practice and practice models. One example of an intradisciplinary model was designed to serve older adults living independently in a rural community. The wellness center's financial base included a federal contact, fee for service, donations, support from the local university, and, eventually, billing third-party payers (64). Interdisciplinary group practice is more complex in some respects and simpler in others. It is also realistic in a time of knowledge explosion, advances in therapies and technology, and limits on what any one health care professional is prepared to do, or should do given her/his educational preparation and experience. Advanced practice nurses are skilled in establishing collaborative practices with other health care professionals. In undertaking a collaborative relationship, it is important to agree on the contributions expected from each member based on competence, knowledge and skills, and the benefits of collaboration on the quality and outcomes of patient care. Benefits to each team member need to be explored as well. Developing means for regular communication, ways of resolving differences, and guidelines for helping each other will help the collaboration be successful (62). In one interdisciplinary collaborative practice, team members set aside time each week to discuss problems, find solutions, and communicate with one another.

Developing a written collaborative practice agreement is a means to assure that as many issues as possible are discussed ahead of time and, also, seeing these in writing can help all parties understand their roles and responsibilities (45, 65). One author has divided these issues into three categories: definitions, specific clinical issues, and business/legal issues. This author also suggests collecting relevant documents as appendixes to the practice agreement, e.g., documents such as the state nurse practice act, prescriptive authority, and rules and regulations governing advanced practice nurses, clinical practical guidelines or protocols, peer review materials, and so on (45).

If you are joining the practice of another provider, you will enjoy the advantages of moving into an established office with a caseload already in place. In group practice, financial commitments can vary widely. You may be asked to contribute to operating costs at a percentage based on income generated, at a fixed rate, or at a level allowing you to "buy into" the practice. If you become a salaried employee of a group, your role in decision making will be significantly different than if you are a partner. That is an important distinction to make when considering the various alternatives for financial arrangements. It is impossible to become an owner or shareholder in an incorporated practice or enter into a business partnership. Since regulations vary from state to state with regard to interdisciplinary professional corporations or partnerships, it is best to engage the services of an attorney (5, 13). In 1979, California passed a bill permitting registered nurses to own up to 49% of shares in professional medical corporations (16). Since that time, many other states have followed their example.

You might also choose to enter into a collaborative relationship with other providers whereby you each contribute to overhead expenses but keep separate business accounts, billing procedures, fee schedules, and so on. You then could set up protocols for consultation or collaboration with the others and they with you on a fee-for-service, reciprocal or gratis arrangement. You and another provider might also wish to consider contracting with each other for services on the basis of a guaranteed income or on a fee-for-service basis. A nurse and a physician might contract for the services of a nutritionist, or a physician might contract for the services of an advanced practice nurse, or vice versa. In some states where advanced practice nurses must have a supervising or collaborating physician, creating a formal contractual arrangement may be one way of fulfilling this legal requirement. For example, a group practice of nurse-midwives might contract with an obstetrician/gynecologist for back-up.

Thus, as can be seen, there are several interesting arrangements to consider when preparing to set up a collaborative practice (17). Gathering data and assessing each option will enable you to make a decision based on a thorough understanding of the advantages and disadvantages of each. There are also numerous examples in the literature of nurses in collaborative practices as entrepreneurs, exploring and creating new roles and serving new markets (15, 18).

New Models of Entrepreneurial Practice
Many entrepreneurial models for advanced practice have emerged since Lucille Kinlein began her independent practice. It might be argued that, in some ways, nurses have always found ways to be entrepreneurs, for there are numerous examples such as Jane Hitchcock working independently teaching public health nursing in schools of nursing (19). The advent of advanced practice as nurse anesthetics, nurse-midwives, clinical nurse specialists, and nurse

practitioners meant new opportunities for nurse entrepreneurs. Changes in legislation and rules and regulations affecting advanced practice nurses, consumer acceptance, access to designation on provider panels of managed care organizations, and accumulating evidence that advanced practice nurses help to control costs, all suggest that nurse-managed centers may thrive in the twenty-first century (77).

Consultation (78, 79) and health education, maternity fitness, home care services for special patient groups including persons with AIDS, endstage renal disease, new babies and children with chronic care needs, stress management, postpartum depression, nurse managed centers, private case management, and media services are only some of the innovative businesses begun by nurses prepared for advanced practice (15, 18, 21). The term intrapreneurial practice has been applied to nurses organizing as a company to provide nursing services to agencies and institutions or practicing as affiliates of existing hospitals, in community based nursing centers, in independent practice in inpatient settings and in private case management (20, 22, 29, 66). Several resources for nurses considering entrepreneurial roles are included in the bibliography.

At a time "when the walls that divide inpatient, outpatient, primary, tertiary, and community care are coming down" (73, p. 117), advance practice nurses should be open to exploring new models for practice, whether as salaried employees, in collaborative practices, as contractors for managed care systems, or in independent nurse-managed practices. The economic aspects of advanced practice roles will become even more complex under managed care systems, integrated and seamless systems of care delivery, and consolidation of third-party payers. Advanced practice nurses need to understand all the reimbursement systems and how these affect their practice.

Third-Party Reimbursement
Several attempts to bring about change in reimbursement policies to nurses have been made, the earliest in 1948 (25), and some of these efforts have been successful and will be described here. However,

present reimbursement schemes in some states still not only preclude third-party reimbursement for nurses and other non-physician providers, but also limit access for patients who are unable to pay out-of-pocket. Thus, many consumers are not able to have direct access to nursing services. The present chaos has created bidding wars among third-party payers for employee plans and among hospitals for managed care contracts, created networks of services and panels (sometimes all-physician) of providers, has launched considerable debate on who can be designated a primary care provider, and sometimes leaves the decision to grant or deny services to a business person (26, 80). As we continue to move toward large managed care systems and integrated care systems, all health care providers may become either employees or contractors or both under such systems. In the continuing chaos, however, it is still germane to discuss third-part reimbursement schemes and how they affect advanced practice nurses.

Recognizing the importance of developing new models for reimbursement for providers, Congress, in the Social Security Amendments of 1972 (P.L. 92-603), authorized experiments and demonstration projects focused on methods and amounts of reimbursement for services performed by independent providers. Thus the Physician Extender Reimbursement Study was launched (27). While nurses may react unfavorably to being classified as "physician extenders," the concept of independent reimbursement is critical.

In 1982, direct reimbursement for nurse-midwives was authorized through Medicaid (33). Since that time, the federal government has allowed states to administer Medicaid within broad general guidelines. Often this means only policy change for nurses to get direct reimbursement (34). The Department of Defense previously adopted a policy for direct payment for nurse-midwives through CHAMPUS, its program for the health care of dependents (31). In 1980, Maryland became the first state to provide direct reimbursement for nurses and other non-physician providers through all health insurance (35). Maryland had previously passed bills allowing reimbursement for nurse-midwives and nurse practitioners (36, 37, 38).

The Rural Health Clinic Services (RHCS) Act of 1977 (P.L. 95-

210) authorizes Medicare and Medicaid payments to qualified rural health clinics for the services of nurse practitioners (39). Clinics must apply to become certified in order to be eligible for reimbursement. In 1988, changes in the Act rekindled interest in use of its provisions to assist rural hospitals and health clinics (40), and in the Omnibus Budget Reconciliation Act of 1989, new RHCS provisions enhanced its potential for advanced practitioners (41). In 1987, the Federal Employees Health Care Freedom of Choice Act was passed by Congress. This bill mandates direct third-party reimbursement to nurses, nurse practitioners, nurse-midwives, and several other non-physician health care providers under the Federal Employees Health Benefits Program. This bill has important implications for nurses in advanced practice (46, 47).

In 1997, Public Law 105-33 was enacted providing Medicare Part B coverage and direct payment for services provided by nurse practitioners and clinical nurse specialists if those services would be reimbursable if provided by a physician without regard for geographic area or setting. (Previous legislation allowed this coverage but only in rural areas and, for some services, only in nursing homes). This law went into effect on January 1, 1998, and allows reimbursement at 85% of the physician rate. The original legislation stipulated that the advanced practice nurse must be providing care in collaboration with a physician and also mandated master's preparation for these nurses (28, 85). When advanced practice nurses raised questions about these requirements, the Health Care Financing Administration (HCFA) took under advisement proposals to modify the definition of collaboration and to grandfather in certificate prepared nurses. The wording of the requirement for collaboration has been modified and will make practice in states without legislated collaboration requirements easier (86). Further tinkering by HCFA will undoubtedly continue, as the rules and regulations leave many questions for providers (87, 88).

While this legislation was a significant victory for advanced practice nurses, it has raised critical questions about achieving provider status and acquiring the provider credentials necessary to receive reimbursement. Medicare provides benefits for its enrolled patients either through a managed care organization (MCO) or on a fee-for-service arrangement with a provider. If the advance practice nurse is a contractor with a MCO, she or he must apply to be admitted to the provider panel for that MCO (48). As a contractor, an advanced practice nurse could conceivably have patients in the practice whose coverage is with any number of MCOs that do business in that state and accept Medicare enrollees. Thus credentialing for the provider become cumbersome. Additionally, to receive approval for reimbursement on a fee-for-service basis, the advanced practice nurse must apply to be a Medicare provider. As employees of rural federally designated rural health clinics, federally qualified health centers, and health maintenance organizations, the facility rather than the provider receives the payment for the Medicare enrollee (84).

Because documentation for reimbursement is generated out of current procedural terminology (CPT) codes developed by the American Medical Association and commonly used by third-party payers for use in reimbursement claims and by the International Classification of Diseases, 9th revision (referred to as ICD-9) for medical diagnoses, advanced practice nurses who will be billing directly as well as those whose facilities do the billing have to have sufficient mastery of these two systems to facilitate the paperwork necessary for reimbursement (48).

To facilitate identity and mobility of health care providers, HCFA will be imposing national identification numbers. This single number will replace the multiple numbers physicians, nurse practitioners, and physician assistants typically have and will also replace the separate Medicare, Medicaid, Blue Cross/Blue Shield, and professional licensure numbers (89). Other providers such as registered nurses, physical therapists, and so on, will be billed under the provider who delegated the care to them pursuant to the Medicare reimbursement rules and regulations (90).

Federal legislation allows selected advanced practice nurses to apply for reimbursement for services to Medicaid recipients. Since Medicaid is a jointly administered federal-state program, each state has to pass legislation allowing advanced practice nurses to apply for provider status and bill that state's Medicaid program directly (32, 42). Achieving Medicaid provider status is a cumbersome process. Direct application for a provider number must be made through the state Medicaid agency. Within managed care organizations, advanced practice nurses must apply and be accepted on the provider panel for that MCO (48). If more than one MCO accepting Medicaid patients exists in a state and an advanced practice nurse cares for persons enrolled in these, the advanced practice nurse must apply to each one. Some Medicaid patients are also covered by indemnity insurers that pay health care providers on a per-procedure basis. To be eligible for this reimbursement, advanced practice nurses have to inquire of each indemnity company whether it requires a provider number and, if so, must apply for this credential in order to bill (42, 48).

Clarification of the complex rules and regulations for Medicare reimbursement and the imposition of CPT codes and ICD-9 for diagnosis mandate that advanced practice nurses have up-to-date information. Websites are helpful as they can be updated daily if necessary. If we are to benefit from legislation that is increasingly permissive for direct reimbursement for the care we provide, we have to assume responsibility for knowing how to access this reimbursement in an expeditious manner with as few denials as possible and within the law as it currently is written and interpreted.

By 1999, 47 states had passed legislation recognizing some form of third-party reimbursement for nurse practitioners. Some states which have passed legislation specify reimbursement for nurse practitioners, some for nurse-midwives, and some for a variety of nurses in advanced practice positions. In 32 states, clinical nurse specialists are eligible for third-party reimbursement, as are nurse-midwives in 33 states and anesthetists in 38 (42). Third-party reimbursement through Blue Cross/Blue Shield and private insurance carriers is also available to nurses in some states (48). And in most states, some advanced practice nurses in specified categories are receiving direct reimbursement from private insurance companies, although there are states in which no legislative authority exists as yet (42). In fact, private insurers can establish their own policies, so legislative change is often not necessary.

It seems evident that if nurses are to achieve full recognition under third-party reimbursement plans, both federal and private, we must be politically active (24, 80, 85, 91, 92). We must be in the forefront of health policy decision-making and utilize the power inherent in the numbers of health care providers we represent when negotiating to be on provider panels and for recognition as primary care providers. To paraphrase Taylor, we must be recognized as essential providers of care (60).

Benefits and Cost Effectiveness of Advanced Practice Nursing
In a compelling article, Safriet argued that advanced practice nurses are cost-effective, deliver high quality care to needy patients, and that limitations on scope of practice, third-party reimbursement and prescription writing privileges should be eliminated. Her thorough review of these issues provides a useful tool for several purposes: legislative and policy change at the state level; health care reform at the state and federal levels; negotiating positions in employing agencies, institutions, and group practices; and documenting the cost effectiveness and benefits of advanced practice nurses (49). Since that article was published in 1992, legal and regulatory barriers have been eliminated in many states. In 1998, Safriet contended that the new challenges have been created by the competitive character of the health care marketplace, integrated care systems, and schemes for contracting with care providers or creating panels of providers (80).

Numerous models have been proposed and tested for assessing the cost-effectiveness and benefits of nurses in a variety of advanced practice roles (50, 51, 52, 53, 54). Some of these have clinical utility as part of quality improvement programs. They also help nurses to assess how they spend their time, the revenues they generate for the agency or practice, and how they might alter their activities to prevent burnout. Incorporating such data collection as part of roles in advanced practice will help to assure that advanced practitioners are not forgotten in the current health care chaos.

Salaries and Employment of Nurses in Advanced Practice

Knowing the salary and employment characteristics of nurses in advanced practice is useful in negotiating for a position and, in particular, in instituting an advanced practice role in an agency, institution or practice where there has not been an advanced practice nurse before. There are several sources of data on such issues. (See Bibliography). Several specialty organizations and state nurse practitioner groups have conducted and published salary surveys. The American Nurses Association collects data on characteristics of employment of nurses in advanced practice roles. Several interdisciplinary organizations and publications also conduct salary surveys (56, 82, 83).

A survey of salaries for nurse-midwives revealed that experience and full-time salaried work are more important salary determinants than are hours worked including on-call time (55). The mean salary was $57,000 (56). One 1999 study of nurse practitioner salaries and benefits revealed a range of base salaries from $50,000 to $105,000 (56). Salaries for clinical nurse specialists range from $45,000 to $73,000, and for nurse anesthetists the average annual salary is $79,600 (56). The mean for nurse anesthetists in another survey was $83,000 (76). Data from 1995 yielded the following median salaries: nurse anesthetist, $80,469, and nurse practitioner, $49,200 (82). Region of the country and academic preparation also affect salaries as does the influence of managed care's share of the market. Nurses in advanced practice should learn to negotiate for salary and benefits commensurate with the value of their services.

Since other health care professionals are marketing their services to the public, it is clear that if we are to succeed in a competitive health care arena, we must learn to market ourselves. Strategies can include hosting talk shows on health care issues, writing a column or an editorial for a local newspaper, generating advertisements, news releases, fact sheets, brochures, newsletters and direct mailings for consumers, and conducting marketing surveys (see Chapter 12), personal interviews in the media, speeches to lay groups, and developing a profile of providers who might be potential competitors as well as referents (58, 59). Marketing includes selling ourselves to other health care providers and to managed care systems as well as to the public. Our relationships with patients will demonstrate what we have to offer. There are numerous resources in the literature on marketing strategies, and there are classes and courses on the subject offered at colleges, universities, and adult education programs (59). (See Online Resources, page 153, for websites.)

Nurse-Managed Practice

When Lucille Kinlein hung out her shingle announcing her independent nursing practice, she was unorthodox in more than one respect. Nurses have long been relegated to economically dependent roles within the context of a free enterprise health care delivery system. Caught up in such a tradition, nurses have been slow to enter the economic world of the twentieth century as we enter the twenty-first. Kinlein was a risk-taker in an economic sense, and those who followed her example were willing to brave the economic uncertainties of the new role.

One of the hazards inherent in nurse-managed practice is economic uncertainty. The public is unaccustomed to paying nurses directly for their services. Furthermore, third-party reimbursement mechanisms for nurses are still not well-developed in every state, so in some settings and some states nurses must rely on associations with physicians or on special circumstances such as rural health center status in order to be directly reimbursed, or special populations such as nursing home residents or recipients of Medicare or Medicaid. Because of reimbursement, some types of advanced practice nurses may be more able than others to set up nurse-managed practices.

Planning for a Nurse-Managed Practice

Launching an independent practice requires far more than developing a philosophy of care, a plan to implement that philosophy in practice, and means for evaluation (1). A nurse-managed practice requires thoughtful planning for its financial as well as for the operational aspects and creation of the caregiving team (13).

Acquiring business skills is very helpful for the nurse who is setting up a practice. Short courses, workshops, and college classes on business are available (2). Lots of online resources exist as well (see end of chapter). Little has yet been done to incorporate courses in business and economics into undergraduate or graduate nursing programs (3), although current programs include more information about the economic aspects of advanced practice roles. When a nurse-managed practice is a faculty practice, help may be available through the university's school of management or business office. In order to maximize the potential of nurses prepared to practice as independent providers, perhaps these nurses need "some basic training in being an entrepreneur"(3). Before launching a nurse-managed practice, a business plan is essential (78).

Assessment. Simplistic as it may sound, setting up a nurse-managed practice should follow the steps of the nursing process. First, you will need to spend a considerable amount of time assessing the needs of your proposed target patient population, formulating and/or articulating the philosophy, objectives, and scope of your practice, preparing protocols, collecting information on how you will fit in and work with other health care providers, and surveying possible locations. In business language, this is a survey of the industry and a market analysis (78).

Some of the components of the assessment process (philosophy and scope of practice, community needs, market analysis, and interdisciplinary relationships) are addressed in other chapters. Here we will concentrate on the business and economic aspects. Creating the business plan will include gathering information on reimbursement for services, the costs of renting space, telephone service, advertising, any necessary equipment to rent or purchase, disposable or reusable supplies, record-keeping materials, handling of hazardous wastes, security, and various means for financing a small business.

Financial Planning. An important component of a business plan is the financial plan. Your assessment will provide you with the data on start-up costs. Beginning a nurse-managed practice can cost up to several thousand dollars, but it can be done on shoestring with careful planning (10). Academic nursing centers often began on a shoestring with considerable support from their parent schools of nursing and grants. To survive in the twenty-first century, they need to have sound business plans (11). Allowing for inflation, it is probable that you can plan on at least several hundred dollars as an absolute minimum (see Table 8.2). In addition to the actual costs involved in equipping and supplying an office, getting office supplies and a telephone, advertising, and so on, it is imperative to plan for expenses that will be ongoing, such as rent, until you can expect the

Table 8.2 Start-up Costs for a Practice*

Rent for first and last months
Deposit on rental
Stationery supplies and office forms
Telephone installation and deposit (one or more lines)
Telephone answering machine or answering service
Incorporation fees
Equipment for office and examining room − probably include
  computer, copy machine, fax machine
Laboratory equipment including microscope, Glucometer®
Supplies for examinations and record keeping
Advertising: brochures, ads, mailings, newsletter, business
  cards, signs, yellow pages, website
Utility deposits and/or meter installation fees
Fees such as licensure
Any decorating or remodeling costs
Malpractice insurance
Attorney, accountant, architect fees
Incidentals: petty cash, coffee, tea bags, cups, toilet paper, paper
  towels, etc.
Checking account − cost of having checks printed, any service
  charges
Educational materials for patients
Computer and/or word processor supplies
Financing costs
Contingency fund (minimum of 5% of budget)

* Adapted from Dalton (4), Pearson (9), and Nichols and Nichols (10)

practice to be self-supporting (9) (see Table 8.3). If you plan to devote full time to the practice, you also need to plan for your living costs until the practice generates an income for you over and above business costs (2) (see Table 8.4).

Table 8.3 Operating Expenses

Rent or mortgage
Utilities: light, heat, water
Telephone, online service
Telephone answering service or voicemail, if needed
Maintenance: cleaning services and cleaning supplies and
   equipment; maintenance cost for office equipment; hazardous waste
   disposal
Disposables: office supplies, examination room and laboratory
   supplies, miscellaneous such as coffee, tea, etc.
Laboratory fees
Advertising: ads, brochures, newsletter, yellow pages, business cards
Laundry services – lab coats, scrub suits, towels, gowns, table
   covers
Malpractice insurance and other insurance fees such as theft, fire, and
   business taxes; Social Security
Accountant fees
Postage
Checks: service for checking account
Duplication of records for referral

When you have determined the initial costs and business and personal expenses for the first few months of practice, it is time to evaluate your assets and debits to determine if you can afford to go into private practice. If your anticipated start-up costs exceed your resources, other sources of funds must be sought. Consider small business loans. The assistance of a banker or financial officer versed in the economic aspects of starting a small business can be invaluable. Other sources of funds include: personal loans, private investment companies, government lending programs, small

Table 8.4. Personal Expenses*

Rent, condominium fees and/or mortgage and taxes
Food
Insurance: health, life, property
Car insurance and taxes, licenses, operating expenses
Upkeep of home
Clothing
Utilities: gas, water, electricity; oil, wood or coal (for heat)
Telephone
Any outstanding loan or credit payments
Taxes: federal, state, local
Medical, dental expenses
Dues, subscriptions to journals, licensure and registration fees,
　　travel to professional meetings, maintenance of licensure,
　　prescription authority and certification, continuing education courses
Recreation: movies, travel, plays, concerts, vacations, eating out
Miscellaneous: newspapers, cosmetics, OTC drugs, laundry,
　　cleaning supplies, personal hygiene products, postage, gifts,
　　educational expense
Pets: care and feeding

* Adapted from Edmunds (2). Figure for all persons whose sole income will come from the practice or proportion by percent of income from the practice.

business investment companies, business development companies, loan companies, and equipment finance companies (13). Since interest charges, fees, loan terms, and collateral statements can be very complex, it is prudent to seek professional advice.

Once you have financing for your business, the next step is to plan short-and long-term budgets. Predictions as to financial viability must be based on the experiences of others, so search the literature and talk with health care providers in your area. Be realistic and conservative in your projections for break-even and profit points.

Budget planning necessitates fee setting (7). Fees reflect how you value your services. At the same time, they must be realistic in relation to the means of your target population and in line with the fees charged by other providers. Some nurses choose to have sliding scale fees. Your method of fee collection will also affect income. If the fees are paid at the time of service, you will eliminate the time lag between the visit and payment, and your bookkeeping will be easier. Deferred billing may sometimes be a reasonable approach to assure that service is not denied to those who need it. Persons on fixed incomes may find a flexible payment scheme helpful (7). It is realistic to plan on some uncollectible fees. If you contract with third parties such as a managed care system, Medicaid, Medicare, or private insurers, be prepared for a lot of paperwork when billing them.

The next step, unless you have some expertise in bookkeeping and accounting, is to seek the services of an accountant. You will need to set up a bookkeeping system to account for all income and output. Some good and inexpensive computer programs are available. You may need federal and state identification numbers for reporting purposes. Some cities and also some states require a business license.

If you decide to employ a receptionist or an assistant of some sort, you will need to develop payroll protocols and comply with regulations for tax withholding and social security payments. It is best to have completely separate bank accounts and bookkeeping for your business and personal accounts (5). Once you are actually using the bookkeeping and patient record systems you planned so carefully, you may find they are too cumbersome or time consuming or incomplete. With the best planning in the world, systems cannot be perfected until they are actually used.

Business Arrangements. When selecting a name for your practice, consider one that will convey who and what you are, one that people will remember, one that is not offensive in any way or that will put people off, and one that does not duplicate the names of other groups or individuals. You may want to incorporate. In that event, your attorney will assist you in researching names of corporations already in use in the state. Incorporating will protect your personal assets from malpractice suits (7, 13). After naming your practice, visit several printing services for estimates and have business cards, stationery, and perhaps brochures prepared. In planning for telephone services, inquire about advertising in the yellow pages, answering services, voice mail services, business rates, and any deposit or installation fees required. Consider creating a website for your practice. Once you have a location and have made it functional, you will need to advertise for patients. Advertising requires a lot of public relations work. You may choose to advertise in the local paper. A mailing of brochures to prospective groups or organizations can be helpful. You will need to make yourself known to other providers: health care professionals, clergy, social service agencies, senior citizen's centers, childbirth education groups, or whatever is appropriate to your practice (15). You may also want to consider being a referral provider for one or more managed care systems.

Selecting a Site. The location for your practice may be critical to its success. Unless you plan a practice which encompasses only home visits, you will need space in which to interview and perhaps examine your patients. You may even need an office out of which to operate your home care business, especially if you have employees and equipment (15). Some advanced practice nurses have been able to convert one room into an adequate office and consulting room, either in their apartment or private residence. It is important to check zoning laws, however, so as not to violate any regulations. If it is not feasible to use space in a private residence, or if the location is not central to your target population, you will have to look for space elsewhere since access for your patients is of utmost importance.

When looking for space, consider proximity to public transportation and available parking space. Choose a building that has an elevator and is accessible to those with disabilities (4, 5). Consider whether the neighborhood is a safe one for you and your patients, and whether it is one that will attract patients for you. If your target population is older people, consider locating near a senior citizen's housing project or senior center (81). Academic nursing centers are often housed in college or university facilities. If it is a low-income population, select a site in such a neighborhood. It may be possible to share an office suite with other providers. Perhaps a local dentist has two or more offices and would be willing to rent one to you. You may also consider group, collaborative, or cooperative practice with other nurses or with physicians or other health care providers. The amount of space you anticipate needing is an important consideration. Will you require a waiting area? Will you need an office and an examining room? A bathroom is probably a necessity, even if it is shared with other tenants in the building.

Rent and the terms of the lease are the next considerations. Assess the rent in light of the security deposit required and your ability to carry the costs until your practice is sufficiently established to cover expenses. It is wise to have an attorney review the lease for you (5).

Once you have secured a place, you will need to equip and furnish it. Unless you are fortunate enough to be renting a furnished suite, joining an established group practice, or can make arrangements to buy out a previous tenant or another practice, you need to assess the costs of making your office functional.

Office and waiting room furniture and accessories such as lamps, rugs, and curtains are often available in secondhand stores or even from your own household, family, and friends. A computer is one item you may need to buy new. If you require examining room equipment, costs can escalate quickly. Comparison shop, check sources for used equipment, check into borrowing equipment, and do a thorough search before you decide on new equipment. A new examining table can cost hundreds of dollars, examination stools and lamps can cost up to a hundred or more dollars each, and miscellaneous equipment such as a side cabinet, otoscope, ophthalmoscope, eye chart, tuning forks, sphygmomanometer, and stethoscope are all expensive. Be sure to include costs of disposable items such as tongue blades, paper for the examining table, drapes for patients (some nurses in advanced practice have made their own washable table covers, johnny gowns, and drapes), and office and record-keeping supplies. If you will be using equipment that can be resterilized, how will you accomplish this? Will you need laundry services of any sort? If you require laboratory services, these must be arranged, and it is possible that you may encounter difficulties in doing so if your practice is exclusively nurses, although such barriers are falling as laboratory services have become profit-making independent businesses (6). Can you meet new Centers for Disease Control (CDC) and Occupational Safety and Health Administration (OSHA) regulations for yourself, any employees, and for handling hazardous waste? Do you need security arrangements if, for example, your nurse-managed center offers first trimester abortions?

Evaluation. Once your office is ready, your advertising under way, and your bookkeeping systems in place, you are ready to begin. As Lucille Kinlein put it, "I sat back and waited for my first client to come" (6, p. 44). After all the planning and anticipation, the big day has arrived—you have a nurse-managed practice!

Evaluation and quality improvement are important and often neglected aspects of independent practice. These are discussed in detail in Chapter Eleven. Evaluating your practice should be ongoing. It is possible to structure your practice so as to elicit input from nurse peers on a periodic basis. If you are in a group nursing practice, you can get input from one another by holding clinical conferences and perhaps meetings on office management as well (4). Setting regular times for evaluation and review will assure that these meetings occur. Soliciting feedback from patients will help you assess which services they most value, how best to reach the potential patient population, and how to be most responsive to your patients' perceptions of their needs. Furthermore, evaluation, quality improvement, and outcome measures will provide data to support direct third-party reimbursement and contracting with managed care organizations for nurses.

Summary
Clearly, advanced practice nursing is at an economic crossroad. We can content ourselves with being cogs in the giant economic machine of our chaotic health care system or we can seize the power that is rightfully ours as the largest group of professional providers.

If we are to be creators of policy for health care, it is important to strengthen our position by researching the costs of nursing services delivered through nursing models, educating the public on the value of nursing services, soliciting consumer advocacy for nurses, and gaining control of our practice within our work settings (60). To quote Taylor, "It is imperative that we in nursing practice,education, and research be knowledgeable about, prepared for, able to advocate for, and participate in the creation of a preferred future in health care policy and practice" (60, pp. 50-51).

REFERENCES

1. Rew, L. (1988). AFFIRM the role of clinical specialist in private practice. *Clinical Nurse Specialist 2(1):39-43.*
2. Edmunds, M. (1980). Financial planning for independent practice. *The Nurse Practitioner 5:35-36, 38.*
3. Simms, E. (1977). Preparation for independent practice. *Nursing Outlook 25:114-118.*
4. Dalton, J.B. (1985). Guide to private practice office planning. *The Nurse Practitioner 10(5):43-44, 47, 56.*
5. Jacox, A.K. & Norris, C.M. (Eds.) (1977). *Organizing for Independent Nursing Practice.* New York: Appleton-Century-Crofts. p. 127.
6. Kinlein, M.L. (1977). *Independent Nursing Practice with Clients.* Philadelphia: J.B. Lippincott. p. 37.
7. Lanza, M.L. (1996). Money: Personal issues affect professional practice. *Clinical Nurse Specialist 10(6):310-317.*
8. RN fights for title in phone directory. (1981). *American Journal of Nursing 81:265.*
9. Pearson, L.J. (1986). Nancy Dirubbo: Fighting for the rights of NPs in private practice. *The Nurse Practitioner 11(9):52, 57-58, 62.*
10. Nichols, J.S. & Nichols, R.E. (1990). How to start a practice on a shoestring. *Journal of American Academy of Nurse Practitioners 2(3):129-131.*
11. Holman, E.J. & Bransletter, E. (1997). An academic nursing clinic's financial survival. *Nursing Economic$ 15(5):248-252.*
12. Starck, P.L. (1995). Health care reform in '95: Six problems APNs must address. *American Journal of Nursing 95(1):16E-16F, 16H.*
13. Mastrangelo, R. (1993). The challenge and rewards of independent practice. *Advance for Nurse Practitioners 1(4):13-15.*
14. Thomas, C. (1986). How to join and participate in a medical corporation. *The Nurse Practitioner 11(9):64, 67, 71.*
15. Mastrangelo, R. (1994). Getting into the business of . . . home care. *Advance for*

Nurse Practitioners 2(9):24-26.
16. California RNs can now own shares in joint RN-MD professional practices. (1979). *American Journal of Nursing 79:2074.*
17. Wille, R. & Frederickson, K.C. (1981). Establishing a group private practice in nursing. *Nursing Outlook 29:522-524.*
18. Clark, L. & Quinn, J. (1988). The new entrepreneurs. *Nursing and Health Care 9(1):7-15.*
19. Kaufman, M., Hawkins, J.W., Higgins, L.P. & Friedman, A.H. (1988). *Dictionary of American Nursing Biography.* New York: Greenwood Press.
20. American Nurses Association. (1987). The nursing center: Concept and design. Kansas City, MO: ANA.
21. Wallace, B. Nurses move outside traditional roles. *NAACOG Newsletter, June, 1987.*
22. Boyer, D.C. & Martinson, D.J. (1990). Intrapreneurial group practice. *Nursing & Health Care II(1):29-32.*
23. Mahoney, D.F. (1988). An economic analysis of the nurse practitioner role. *The Nurse Practitioner 13(3):44-45, 48-50, 52.*
24. Timmons, G. & Ridenour, N. (1994). Legal approaches to the restraint of trade of nurse practitioners: Disparate reimbursement patterns. *Journal of the American Academy of Nurse Practitioners 6:55-59.*
25. Jennings, C.P. (1977). Third party reimbursement and the nurse practitioner. *The Nurse Practitioner 2:11-13.*
26. Shindul-Rothschild, J. & Gordon, S. (1994). Single-payer versus managed competition: Implications for nurses. *Journal of Nursing Education 33(5):198-207.*
27. Morris, S.B. & Smith, D.B. (1976). The Physician Extender Reimbursement Study. The Diffusion of Physician Extenders (Working Paper No. 1). Washington, DC: U.S. Social Security Administration, Office of Research and Statistics.
28. Minarik, P. (1998). Medicaid and Medicare reimbursement: New law and new legislation. *Clinical Nurse Specialist 12(2):83-84.*
29. Campbell, J.L., Brandel, S.M., Daramola, O.I., Postallian, M.A., Dorris, G.A. & Provenzano, L.J. (1995). Thee advanced practice model: Inpatient collaborative practices. *Clinical Nurse Specialist 9:175-179.*
30. Bakker, D.J. & Vincensi, B.B. (1995). Economic impact of the CNS practitioner role. *Clinical Nurse Specialist 9:50-53.*
31. ANA backs direct reimbursement to nurse-midwives under Medicare. (1979). *American Journal of Nursing 79:2070.*4
32. Doty, R.E. (1996). Illinois Medicaid reimbursement policy for nurse practitioners. *Clinical Nurse Specialist 10:116-119.*
33. Nurse-midwives win direct reimbursement under Medicaid. (1982). *American Journal of Nursing 82:1335.*
34. Pearson, L.J. (1990). The issue of third-party reimbursement — advice for nurse practitioners from a national expert. *The Nurse Practitioner 15(3):46-47.*
35. Maryland is first state to require third-party payment for nurses. (1980). *American Journal of Nursing 80:7.*
36. CNM services are reimbursable in Maryland. (1978). *American Journal of*

Nursing 78:1143-1178.
37. Griffith, H.M. (1982). Strategies for direct third-party reimbursement for nurses. *American Journal of Nursing 82:408-411.*
38. Goldwater, M. (1982). From a legislator: Views on third-party reimbursement for nurses. *American Journal of Nursing 82:411-414.*
39. *Rural Health Clinic Services.* (1979). Hyattsville, MD: Department of Health, Education, and Welfare. p. 1.
40. Rural Health Clinics Act offers revenue benefits. (1988) *The Nurse Practitioner 13(8):64, 66.*
41. Wasem, C. (1990). The Rural Health Clinic Services Act: A sleeping giant of reimbursement. *Journal of the American Academy of Nurse Practitioners 2(2):85-87.*
42. Pearson, L.J. (1999). Annual update of how each state stands on legislative issues affecting advanced nursing practice. *Nurse Practitioner 24(1):16-83.*
43. Towers, J. (1992). The status of Medicare reimbursement for nurse practitioners. *Journal of the American Academy of Nurse Practitioners 4(3):129-130.*
44. Davis, E.A. (1994). Factors influencing the implementation of the CNS role in a private practice. *Clinical Nurse Specialist 8:42-47.*
45. Sebas, M.B. (1994). Developing a collaborative practice agreement for the primary care setting. *Nurse Practitioner 19(3):49-51.*
46. Knox, J.T. (1988). Direct reimbursement to nurse practitioners: The importance of the Federal Employees Health Care Freedom of Choice Act (H.R. 382). *The Nurse Practitioner 13(11):52-53.*
47. Stallmeyer, J. (1986). Direct reimbursement for NPs under FEHBP. *The Nurse Practitioner 11(6):14,16.*
48. Buppert, C. (1998). Reimbursement for nurse practitioner services. *Nurse Practitioner 23(1):67-81.*
49. Safriet, B.J. (1992). Health care dollars and regulatory sense: The role of advanced practice nursing. *Yale Journal on Regulation 9:417-488.*
50. Gift, A.G. (1992). Determining CNS cost effectiveness. *Clinical Nurse Specialist 6(2):89.*
51. McGrath, S. (1990). The cost-effectiveness of nurse practitioners. *The Nurse Practitioner 15(7):40-42.*
52. Gardner, D. (1992). The CNS as a cost manager. *Clinical Nurse Specialist 6(2):112-116.*
53. Edwardson, S.R. (1992). Costs and benefits of clinical nurse specialists. *Clinical Nurse Specialist 6(3):163-167.*
54. Kearnes, D.R. (1992). A productivity tool to evaluate NP practice: Monitoring clinical time spent in reimbursable patient-related activities. *The Nurse Practitioner 17(4):50, 52, 55.*
55. Lehrman, E. (1992). Findings of the 1990 annual American College of Nurse-Midwives membership survey. *Journal of Nurse-Midwifery 37(1):33-47.*
56. Segal-Isaacson, A. (1999). What will they pay me? A review of salary and benefits data reveals encouraging news of APNs. *Advanced Practice Nurse Sourcebook 1998/9.* Springhouuse, PA: Springhouse.
57. American Nurses Association. (1993). Advanced practice nursing: A new age

in health care. *Nursing Facts.* Washington, DC: Author.
58. Pearson, L.J. (1986). Jo Ann Woodward: Opening channels of communication: Marketing the NP role. *The Nurse Practitioner 11(11):55,59-60,62.*
59. Gardner, K.L. & Weinrauch, D.(1988). Marketing strategies for nurse entrepreneurs. *The Nurse Practitioner 13(5):46, 48-49.*
60. Taylor, D. (1998). Crystal ball gazing: Back to the future. *Advanced Practice Nursing Quarterly 3(4):44-51.*
61. Grabowski, V.M. & Jens, G.P. (1993). The collaborative role of the CNS in support groups. *Clinical Nurse Specialist 77:99-101.*
62. Stichler, J.F. (1995). Professional interdependence: The art of collaboration. *Advanced Practice Nurse Quarterly 1:53-61.*
63. Kopser, K.G., Horn, P.B. & Carpenter, A.D. (1994). Successful collaboration within an integrative practice model. *Clinical Nurse Specialist 8:331-333.*
64. Hawkins, J.W., Igou, J.F., Johnson, E.E. & Utley, Q.E. (1988). An intradisciplinary team in a nurse managed center. *Nursing Management 19(4):58-59, 62, 64.*
65. Henry, P.F. (1995). The nurse practitioner's guide to practice agreements. *Nurse Practitioner Forum 6(1):4-5.*
66. Kelechi, T.J. & Lukas, K.S. (1996). Intrapreneurial nursing: the lower extremity assessment form. *Clinical Nurse Specialist 10:266-274.*
67. Daleiden, A.L. (1993). The CNS as trauma case manager: A new frontier. *Clinical Nurse Specialist 7:295-298.*
68. Lynn-McHale, D.J., Fitzpatrick, E.R. & Shaffer, R.B. (1993). Case management: Development of a model. *Clinical Nurse Specialist 7:299-307.*
69. Crawley, W.D. & Till, A.H. (1995). Case management: More population-based data. *Clinical Nurse Specialist 9:116-120.*
70. Ferraro-McDuffie, A., Chan, J.S.L. & Jerome, A.M. (1993). Communicating the financial worth of the CNS through the use of fiscal reports. *Clinical Nurse Specialist 7:91-97.*
71. Lamb, G.S. & Stempel, J.E. (1994). Nurse case management from the client's point of view: Growing as insider-expert. *Nursing Outlook 42:7-13.*
72. Madden, M.J. & Ponte, P.R. (1994). Advanced practice roles in the managed care environment. *Journal of Nursing Administration 24:56-62.*
73. Cronenwett, L.R. (1995). Molding the future of advanced practice nursing. *Nursing Outlook 43(3):113.*
74. Brubakken, K.M., Janssen, W.R. & Ruppel, D.L. (1994). CNS role in implementation of a differentiated case management model. *Clinical Nurse Specialist 8:69-73*
75. Sherman, J.J. & Johnson, P.K. (1994). CNS as a unit-based case manager. *Clinical Nurse Specialist 8:76-80.*
76. Waugaman, W.R. & Foster, S.D. (1995). CRNAs: An enviable legacy of patient service. *Advanced Practice Nursing Quarterly 1(1):21-28.*
77. Flanagan, L. (1998, October). Nurse practitioners: Growing competition for family physicians? *Family Practice Management, 34-43.*
78. Schulmmeister, L. (1999). Starting a nursing consultation practice. *Clinical Nurse Specialist 13:94-100.*

79. Schulmeister, L. (1999). The challenges of a home-based nursing consultation business. *Clinical Nurse Specialist 13:101-103.*
80. Safriet, B.J. (1998). Still spending dollars, still searching for sense: Advanced practice nursing in an era of regulatory and economic turmoil. *Advanced Practice Nursing Quarterly 3(4):24-33.*
81. Ryan, M.D. (1997). Integrating practice, education, and research: Killing three birds with one stone. *Clinical Excellence for Nurse Practitioners 1: 244-249.*
82. Marcus, C.L. (1997). PA and NP salaries on the rise. *Clinician Reviews 7(2):134-138.*
83. Pulcini, J., Vampola, D., & Fitzgerald, M.A. (1998). NPACE nurse practitioner practice characteristics, salary and benefits survey. *Clinical Excellence for Nurse Practitioners 2(5):300-306.*
84. Buppert, C. (1998). HCFA releases final roles on PA and NP Medicare reimbursement. *Clinician News 2(6):1, 10, 127-28.*
85. Wong, S.T. (1999). Reimbursement for advanced practice nurses (APNs) through Medicare. *Image 31(2):167-173.*
86. Buppert, C. (1999). The power of association. *Nurse Practitioner World News 1, 16.*
87. See regular column by C. Buppert in *Nurse Practitioner World News* for updates and commentaries on HCFA rulings.
88. Sharp, N. (1998). From 'incident to' to telehealth: New federal rules and regulations affect NPs. *Nurse Practitioner 23(8):68-69.*
89. Buppert, C. (1999). PAs/NPs prepare for "enumeration" HCFA to impose national ID numbers. *Clinician News 3(2):1, 7-8, 13.*
90. Price, L.C. & Minarik, P.A. (1998). More on Medicare reimbursement clarification of direct billing and "incident to" billing. *Clinical Nurse Specialist 12:246-249.*
91. Peters, S. (1998). Grassroots glory. Organizing a campaign that works. *Advance for Nurse Practitioners 6(3):51-54.*
92. Public relations campaign under development in Massachusetts. (1997). *Advance for Nurse Practitioners 5:9.*

BIBLIOGRAPHY

American Nurses Association. (1998). *Managed care: Nursing's blueprint for action.* *

Attenborough, R. (1997). The Canadian health care system: Development, reform, and opportunities for nurses. *Journal of Obstetric, Gynecologic, and Neonatal Nursing 26:229-234.*

Bendell, A. (1997). Health care in the 1990s: Changes in health care delivery models for survival. *Journal of Obstetric, Gynecologic, and Neonatal Nursing 26:212-216.*

Bower, K.A. (1992). *Case Management by Nurses.* *

Buerhaus, P.I. (1998). Medicare payment for advance practice nurses: What are the research questions? *Nursing Outlook 46(4):151-153.*

Earn What You're Worth: A Nurse's Guide to Better Compensation. 1989.*

Flanagan, L. (1995). *What You Need to Know about Today's Workplace: A Survival Guide.* *

Glassman, P.A., Jaconson, P.D. & Asch, S. (1997). Medical necessity and defined coverage benefits in the Oregon health plan. *American Journal of Public Health 87:1053-1058.*

Hamric, A.B. (1998). Using research to influence the regulatory process. *Advanced Practice Nursing Quarterly 4(3):44-50.*

Henry, J.K. (1997). Community nursing centers: Models of nurse managed care. *Journal of Obstetric, Gynecologic, and Neonatal Nursing 26:224-228.*

Lugo, N.R. (1997). Nurse-managed corporate employee wellness centers. *Nurse Practitioner 22(4):104-113.*

May, C.A., Schraeder, C. & Britt, T. (1997). *Managed Care and Case Management: Roles for Professional Nursing.* *

Minarik, P. (1997). Medicare reimbursement for nurse practitioners and clinical nurse specialists passes state legislative and regulatory forum II. *Clinical Nurse Specialist 11(6):274-275.*

Minarik, P. (1997). Federal reimbursement clarified: Issue of recognition shifts to the states. *Clinical Nurse Specialist 11(1):12-13.*

Minarik, P. (1997). Opposition to antitrust legislation: Support for Medicaid and Medicare reimbursement. *Clinical Nurse Specialist 11(3):139-140.*

Murphy, P. (1995). *Nursing Centers: The Time Is Now.* New York: National League for Nursing.

Nurse Practitioners—Guide to Evaluation & Management Coding. Rev. ed. (1999). St. Paul, MN: Medical Learning Inc.

Nurse Practitioners and Certified Nurse-Midwives: A Meta-analysis of Processes of Care, Clinical Outcomes, and Cost-effectiveness of Nurses in Primary Care Roles. (1993).*

Pulcini, J. & Fitzgerald, M.A. (1997). NPACE nurse practitioner practice characteristics, salary and benefits: Eastern United States. *Clinical Excellence for Nurse Practitioners 2(3):185-190.*

The Reimbursement Manual: How to Get Paid for Your Advanced Practice Nursing Services. * 1994.

Robinson, K.R. & Griffith, H.M. (1997). Identification of current procedural terminology-coded services provided by family nurse practitioners. *Clinical Excellence for Nurse Practitioners 1(6):397-404.*

Rural/Frontier Nursing: The Challenge to Grow. (1996). *

Sharp, N. (1997). Medicare reimbursement: For NPs, CNSs, MDs and telehealth. *Nurse Practitioner 22(8):143-146.*

Sinclair, B.P. (1997). Advanced practice nurses in integrated health care systems. *Journal of Obstetric, Gynecologic, and Neonatal Nursing 26:217-233.*

Stone, P.W. & Walker, P.H. (1997). Clinical and cost outcomes of a freestanding birth center: A comparison study. *Clinical Excellence for Nurse Practitioners 1(7):456-465.*

Vogel, G. & Doleysh, N. (1994). *Entrepreneuring: A Nurse's Guide to Starting a Business.* 2nd ed. New York: National League for Nursing.

Wurzbach, M.E. (1998). Managed care: Moral conflict for primary health care nurses. *Nursing Outlook 46(2):62-66.*

---

* Publications available from American Nurses Publishing, American Nurses Association, 600 Maryland Avenue SW, Suite 100 West, Washington, DC 20024-2571.

ONLINE RESOURCES

American College of Nurse Practitioners—state by state lists of Medicare carriers and their phone numbers: **www.aanp.org**

Business Hotline: **www.zbizhotline.com**

Business Women's Network: **www.BWN@tpag.com**

Health Care Financing Administration — Medicaid Program: **www.hcfa.gov/medicaid/medsta95.htm**

Health Care Financing Administration — HCFA statistics at a glance: **www.hefa.gov/stats/stathili/htm**

Health Care Financing Administration rules for Medicare reimbursement for NPs: **www.access.gpo.gov/su_docs/aces002.html**

Internal Revenue Service: **www.irs.gov**

Medicare reimbursement for NPs and CNSs: **www.nursing world.or/gova/medreimb.html**

National Association of Female Executives: www.nafe@nafe.com

Nurse Practitioner Support Services (NPSS) database on salaries: **www.nurse.net**

Network Solutions (to create a web page): **www.internic.net**

Women's Connection: **www.women.connect.com**

9

Negotiating an Employment Contract

Introduction
One of the most crucial tasks of the advanced practice nurse is preparing for and negotiating the employment contract. All too often students are so proud — and rightly so — of their accomplishments upon completing a master's program that the process of contract negotiation does not get all the attention it should. So, too, the experienced advanced practice nurse considering a new position needs to consider an employment contract as an opportunity to use skills and knowledge acquired through clinical practice and interactions within one or more care systems to his/her advantage.

Negotiating a "position package" is the synthesis of the entire educational experience and any practice experiences in an advanced practice role. Here the philosophies of nursing and of specialty care must mesh with the reality of the work world. Nursing theory and nursing science must find fruition in a fertile work environment. Assertive techniques and leadership strategies must be put to the crucial test. If the nurse does not "sell" herself/himself during the negotiating process and behaves in a nonassertive, passive manner, future dealings may be impaired.

Developing a Portfolio
The first step in preparing for negotiating a contract is to develop a portfolio. This should include your written philosophies of nursing, advanced practice roles, and specialty care (not for the eyes of the employer but to help you clarify your views so that the negotiations can be dealt with from strength), a resume and, if you are looking for a research or academic job, a CV. In addition, include a written

description of the type of position you are seeking, documents such as licenses, certification, and prescriptive authority, copies of the state nurse practice act and rules and regulations governing advanced practice, and a thoroughly researched paper about the salary you desire. The purpose of a portfolio is to assemble *all* relevant information about one's self in one place. This becomes the source from which current resumes are developed (1, 2, 14).

Philosophies of Nursing, Advanced Practice Roles, and Specialty Care

One of the first steps toward securing the right position with the most favorable conditions is to have thought out and written clearly articulated, succinct philosophies of nursing, advanced practice roles, and specialty care. All advanced practice nurses would surely state that they want to work in a place where the philosophical position is compatible with their own, since philosophical differences are often a source of disenchantment with a position. When that occurs, is it because the nurse has not solidified a philosophy and therefore cannot deal adequately with specific points in the discussion during the employment interview? To clarify such points, the advanced practice nurse should *write out* philosophies of nursing, advanced practice roles, and specialty care.

The philosophy of nursing has to do with issues of independence, autonomy, and professional growth potential within the work setting. Not longer than three pages, it should address the topics of person, environment, health, and nursing as discussed in Chapter 2.

The written philosophy is not meant as a lofty exercise but rather as a translation of basic concepts into the "real world" setting. Reflection on the concept of "person" leads to a variety of questions about the prospective position. Are active participation by the patient and mutual goal setting encouraged? Is equal emphasis placed on psychosocial and physical needs? What are the supports and/or constraints to desired scope of practice in the environment? Does the setting allow the nurse sufficient time for health teaching? How much control does the nurse have in scheduling patients? Is there opportunity to work with families and with other health care professionals? What are the opportunities for advancement? One's philosophy of health also translates into practical concerns. Is the focus of the employing agency geared toward cure, health maintenance, health promotion, or a balance among these three levels of health care? Or is it a for-profit agency, driven by a profit margin and billable units?

A philosophy of advanced practice roles and specialty care, emanating from the general nursing philosophy, should be written next and evaluated for consistency and logic. It is best limited to one page. It should focus on the specifics of the advanced practice roles and specialty care components of health care delivery such as scope of practice, referral network, relationships with other health care professionals, direct and indirect care components, and research.

The Resume

The resume is extremely important since it is most often the first thing a prospective employer evaluates. It summarizes all the pertinent facts about one's background and professional experiences (1) (see Appendix H).

It is important to differentiate between a professional resume and a curriculum vitae. The primary purpose of a resume is to entice an employer to grant an interview for a position. As such, the style and format will vary for different situations (3). Sometimes a different resume must be developed for each position sought.

Basic information, including personal data, educational endeavors, professional credentials (licensure, certification, DEA number and prescriptive authority, Medicare provider number), and professional experience and activities must be included in the resume, but it can be stylized to emphasize the "fit" between your background and the person the employer is seeking or may be encouraged to seek after seeing your resume. The resume can highlight the responsibilities and functions of your previous jobs, thus delineating what you have to offer. In short, the purpose of a resume is to attract the employer's attention and to make him/her anxious to hire you. Your resume is your entree into the work world. You may be a fantastic conversationalist, but you may not get the chance for an interview if your resume does not "sell" you. The cover letter is an extremely important, yet often overlooked, statement about you, and it is what conveys the initial impression to a potential employer (4).

The Curriculum Vitae (CV)

The curriculum vitae, on the other hand, "is a more rigidly prescribed document designated for use in the highly structural world of academe" (3). Since the CV is used almost exclusively for presenting one's qualifications for an academic position, including that of consultant or researcher, it is not modified as is the resume. The CV follows a standard format and should include personal data, education, experience, research, grants, honors and awards, professional memberships, publications, research presentations, and invited papers (5, 18). The CV is a chronicle of scholarly achievements. Articles published in nonprofessional magazines or talks given to community groups, for example, may not be appropriate for the resume but may be very relevant to the CV if a facet of the position sought involves public relations (3, 18) (see Appendix H).

The CV should be prepared and presented if you are seeking an academic or research position. If you desire a clinical position, the resume is the appropriate document to prepare for your portfolio. If the position sought is a joint clinical and academic appointment, you must be prepared to be interviewed by service persons and academics and have both a resume and a CV.

It is not only the content of the CV or resume which is important, but also its style and manner of presentation. Besides knowing the difference between a resume and CV, you should know what to include or exclude within the general categories mentioned earlier. It is to your disadvantage to exclude important information about your experiences and achievements. It is just as serious to "pad" your CV or resume with insignificant or nonprofessional activities.

It is suggested that you prepare a draft copy of your CV or

resume and submit it to a professional agency, or a mentor who is an experienced academician/clinician for feedback before preparing the final document. The college or university from which you received your preparation for advanced practice may offer such assistance as a service to its alumni/ae. Considering the importance of this document to your professional career, this will be time and/or money well spent.

Next, the appearance of the CV or resume must be considered. An unattractive CV or resume will tarnish the image of the most highly qualified scholar/clinician. The CV or resume should be professionally produced on a high-quality computer or word processor and reproduced on sturdy 8 ½ x 11 bond paper. It should contain no typing errors, erasure marks, misspellings, syntax errors, or uneven margins, and should be cleanly typed. A word to the wise: proofread your CV or resume before copies are reproduced or, better yet, have someone else do it. Any errors will reflect upon you, not on your typist. A word processor/computer is immensely helpful and today almost essential in producing a CV/resume as is a laser printer. Many copy centers have services for resumes, and can take a disk copy and produce a professional document that looks like it was typeset.

Often advanced practitioners are reluctant to spend the money to have a CV or resume professionally typed. This is an instance of being penny wise and pound foolish. Fifty to seventy-five dollars spent on this document could be the key to the right job with more money. The same advice holds true for dressing appropriately for the job interview. Appearance, whether it be yours or that of your resume or CV, does make a definite impression on a potential employer and/or interviewer.

The Position Description and the Job Description
Advanced practice nurses often find themselves seeking positions for which there are no established guidelines or parameters. A general position description written by you is another document to be included in your professional portfolio. This document should be

shared with potential employers. The position description specifies your views about your areas of responsibility, qualifications, and functions (6). If you are seeking a position not specifically advertised in a journal or newspaper, for example, then a written statement of what you hope to do and have to offer is a good idea. Advertised positions usually have a job description which has been written by the employing agency. You should definitely ask to see this document if it is available. "The job description is essential because it states the function for which the nursing staff member is held accountable, the performance expectations, and how that contribution is to be measured" (7). A job description serves as a starting point from which to negotiate the specifics of a given position, and it clarifies areas of potential misunderstanding between employer and employee related to anticipated roles and responsibilities (8). You must ascertain that the roles and responsibilities fall within the scope of practice prescribed by professional organizations, standards of care for your specialty promulgated by a professional organization, the state's nurse practice act, and any other legislation pertinent to advanced practice nurses.

Documents

All pertinent documents regarding your professional career should be included in the portfolio for your personal use. Include copies of professional licenses, evidence of certification, transcripts, malpractice insurance policies, and your state's nurse practice act, and rules and regulations governing advanced practice in your state (1, 14). Also include any position description you have developed, data on salaries and benefits, and evaluation tools.

Salary

Last but not least, you need to do some extensive preparation regarding salary requirements *before* going for a position interview. Jacox and Norris present a useful rule of thumb for the determination of salary range (9) as does Bourne (19). It is first necessary to determine the gross income generated by your services. For example, if you see one patient an hour at a charge of $40 per visit, you will generate $1,400 at 35 hours per week or $72,800 per year. Subtract 40 percent for overhead, medical back-up, and consultation costs, and the resulting figure should be within a reasonable salary range. When you do this kind of salary determination it should be easy to overcome the temptation to timidly accept any salary offered by the employer. Facts and figures put you in the driver's seat. You should also be aware of the salary range in the area where you are seeking employment. Salaries may vary greatly with geographic area. The internet can be a valuable source of salary and position information (10, 11). So can annual periodic salary surveys by various professional groups and organizations (16, 17, 20).

The salary figure quoted should be considered in light of the total benefits package and how important it is to you. Fringe benefits such as health insurance, retirement or pension plan, sick leave, holidays, and vacation time can add approximately 50% percent to the base salary (8, 19). A higher salary without fringe benefits may be worth less than a lower one with fringe benefits. Other fringe benefits to consider are tuition reimbursement, certification and licensure costs, DEA license and the cost of prescriptive authority, time off with pay for professional development and the costs of the continuing education programs, malpractice and life and disability insurance, mileage reimbursement, secretarial services including help with publications and research, and reimbursement for necessary equipment. You may also wish to include time for scholarly activities as part of your responsibilities.

Don't forget to consider the process for determining periodic salary increments and the amounts involved. Is a cost of living increase automatically provided? Is there a union to which advanced practice nurses can belong? If so, what are the dues and the specifics of the union contract? Is it a labor union or professional union contract? How is meritorious service rewarded by the employer? What are the methods and processes used for evaluation? Who evaluates you? Has a system of peer review been established? Wolf (8) suggests keeping a record, with cost-benefit analyses, of patients seen and clinical activities such as research projects, for use in the process of on-going salary renegotiation.

Almost every salary is negotiable; even if you aren't negotiating, the employer is. "Low aspirations can actually disqualify you from jobs . . . If you put a small price on yourself, that's about what the employer will think you are worth" (12). Take the initiative and name a high salary. You can always lower your aspirations, but once you have named your rock-bottom salary it is impossible to command a higher price.

Salary negotiations should take place at the end of the interviewing stage. There is a sound rationale behind this timing. "Until the employer has made up his or her mind to hire you, you aren't worth anything to that person. By delaying money talk, you can develop your strengths, communicate your accomplishments, and show how you can meet the other person's needs so that when the time comes to discuss money, you are actually worth more in his/her eyes" (12).

The Position Interview
Much has been written about the position interview and little about the very important steps that prepare one for it. If you have done the preparation, the interview should go smoothly. In addition to the materials in your professional portfolio, explore the agency/institution or practice you are seeking employment from so you are familiar with its characteristics such as: is it for-profit or not-for-profit, who owns it, is it part of a larger care system, what is the administrative structure, who are its patients, and what is the relationship of advanced practice nurses to other providers? Would you be an employee, a shareholder, and to whom would you be answerable? A corporate parent? Community board? Stockholders? Your philosophy will guide the general questions you want to ask of the employer, and you will be prepared to answer any questions asked of you.

The employer's view of person, environment, health, and nursing as well as of advanced practice roles and specialty care must be ascertained and compared to yours to evaluate compatibility. This task is definitely easier when the questions you ask the employer are generated specifically from your philosophy. Areas of essential agreement must be identified first. If there is incompatibility in areas you have identified as crucial to your basic philosophy (such as time for teaching and for illness prevention), negotiations should center around those issues. If agreement is not possible, that may be sufficient reason to terminate the negotiations no matter how attractive other aspects of the position may be.

Assuming that you have had several interviews and that more than one position is basically in tune with your philosophy, you can prioritize the answers of potential employers to the questions you asked them about philosophy by dividing the answers into positive or negative aspects and using these data to help compare one position with another. Since positions are rarely offered outright at the time of an interview, there should be sufficient time to weigh all the factors carefully.

The resume or CV will serve as a concise outline from which you can elaborate about your education and experience. The job description can serve as the specific point of departure for negotiation of specific roles and responsibilities. Your preparation regarding salary and fringe benefits should give you a comfortable range within which to bargain. Be prepared also to meet with a variety of persons during the interview process. These may include the agency administrator, the nurse director, other health care professionals, and staff members, and may occur at different times.

After you've done your homework, proceed with the interviews in a positive manner. Be assertive and put your best foot forward. Dress appropriately and neatly. Look at interviews as learning experiences. Even if you don't accept a position or are not offered one, what you learn from the interview will help you in future interviews.

The final terms of negotiation should be incorporated into a written document to be renegotiated annually. Through the process of prepared negotiation, you will be in the best possible position for career satisfaction, which will benefit both you and your employer.

Autonomy and Accountability

Mauksch identified four critical issues related to the role and practice of advanced practitioners: autonomy, accountability, patient advocacy, and self-actualization (13). Autonomy and accountability are particularly relevant when considering a professional position. As a potential employee, you should carefully consider your position regarding these issues and explore them with potential employers during interviews.

Autonomy and accountability are interrelated and flow logically from one's philosophy. A job must have the potential for both if you are to practice as you were educated to. Autonomy means having a feeling of independence and self-direction which will enable you to be accountable both to yourself and your patients without an intermediary. Autonomy does not mean that you work in isolation without the benefit of medical and/or other health professional consultation and collaboration, but rather that you are free to practice at the maximum potential permitted legally within the scope of nursing practice. Accountability means the assumption of responsibility inherent in the exercise of one's profession.

Summary

Preparing for employment negotiations includes developing written philosophies of nursing, advanced practice roles, and specialty care. A CV or resume should be compiled and professionally prepared. The professional portfolio should also include a position description and related professional documents. An acceptable salary range and fringe benefits should be determined before the interview. The documents prepared for the portfolio serve as guidelines for the interview. This initial negotiation sets the tone for all future relationships with the prospective employer, colleague, or business partner.

REFERENCES

1.   Edmunds, R. (1980). Developing a marketing portfolio. *The Nurse Practitio-*

ner 5:41-46.
2. Crist, P. & Wilcox, B.L. (198). Transition portfolios: Orchestrating our professional competence. *American Journal of Occupational Therapy 52(9):729-736.*
3. Newcomb, J. & Murphy, P.A. (1979). The curriculum vitae—what it is and what it is not. *Nursing Outlook 27:580-583.*
4. Markey, B.T. & Campbell, R.L. (1996). A resume or curriculum vitae for success. *AORN Journal 63(1):192-202.*
5. Van Leunen, M.C. (1978). *A Handbook for Scholars.* New York: Alfred A. Knopf.
6. Edmunds, M. (1979). The position description. *The Nurse Practitioner 4:45-47.*
7. Brockenshire, A. & Hattstaedt, M.J.O. (1980). Revising job descriptions: A consensus approach. *Supervisor Nurse 11:16-20.*
8. Wolf, G.A. (1980). Negotiating an employment contract. *The Nurse Practitioner 5:55, 60.*
9. Jacox, A.K. & Norris, C.M. (1977). *Organizing for Independent Nursing Practice.* New York: Appleton-Century-Crofts.
10. Waxman, K.T. (1998). Marketing your skills outside hospital walls. *Nursing Management 29(8):48-52.*
11. Wheeler, M. (1998). Perspective: The internet—an invaluable career planning and development resource. *Canadian Journal of Nursing Administration 11(1):31-35.*
12. Chastain, D. (1981). How to play your hand for a salary. *New York Times, Oct. 11, Section 12:60.*
13. Mauksch, I.G. (1978). Critical issues of the nurse practitioner movement. *The Nurse Practitioner 3:35-36.*
14. Burgess, S.E. & Meisener, T. (1997). The professional portfolio: An advanced practice nurse job search marketing tool. *Clinical Excellence for Nurse Practitioners 1(7):468-471.*
15. Harper, D.S. (1999). A professional curriculum vitae will open career doors. *Clinical Excellence for Nurse Practitioners 3(1):43-49.*
16. Pulcini, J., Vampola, D. & Fitzgerald, M.A. (1998). NPACE nurse practitioner practice characteristics, salary and benefits survey. *Clinical Excellence for Nurse Practitioners 2(5):300-306.*
17. Marcus, C.L. (1997). PA and NP salaries on the rise. *Clinician Reviews 7(2):134-138.*
18. Hinck, S.M. (1997). A curriculum vitae that gives you a competitive edge. *Clinical Nurse Specialist 11(4):174-177.*
19. Bourne, H. (1998). *A Great Deal! Compensation Negotiation for Nurse Practitioners & Physician Assistants.* Arcata, CA: Heidi Bourne.

20. Segal-Isaacson, A. (1999). What will they pay me? A review of salary and benefits data reveals encouraging news for APNs. *1998/99 Advance Practice Nurse Sourcebook.* Springhouse, PA: Springhouse.

BIBLIOGRAPHY

Aimes, A., Adkins, S., et al. (1992). Assessing work retention issues. *Journal of Nursing Administration 22:37-41.*

Birdi, K. & Allen, C. (1997). Correlates and perceived outcomes of four types of employee development activity. *Journal of Applied Psychology 82(6):845-857.*

Collins, M. (1991). First impressions made in interviews. *The American Nurse 23(3):24.*

Collins, M. (1991). Resume is key to getting a job. *The American Nurse 23(2): 18.*

Dadich, K.A. 1992). Your resume. *Health Care Trends and Transitions 3(2):20-24.*

Fisher, A.B. (1988). If we're so smart, why aren't we rich? *Savvy, August:36-38, 84-86.*

Hahn, M.S. (1995). Writing an effective resume. *Advance for Nurse Practitioners 3(5):53-56.*

Hargadon, J. (1995). Opportunities for health in contracting. *Health Visitor 68(1): 19-20.*

Henry, P. (1995). The nurse practitioner's guide to practice agreements. *Nurse Practitioner Forum 6(1):4-5.*

Hobbs, B.B. (1998). Taking charge of your career. *American Journal of Nursing 98(1):36-40.*

Houlihan, R. (1991). Interviewing tips for the 90's nurse. *Massachusetts Nurse 61(8):4.*

Jones, A.G. (1991). Gaining control of the CNS role through written contracts. *Clinical Nurse Specialist 5(2):101-104.*

Lowis, M. & Sabo, C.E. (1994). Nurse practitioners: Need for and willingness to hire as viewed by nurse administrators, nurse practitioners, and physicians. *Journal of the American Academy of Nurse Practitioners 6(3):113-119.*

McCloskey, J.C. (1990). Two requirements for job contentment: Autonomy and social integration. *Image 22:140-143.*

Mateo, M.A. & Newton, C. (1997). Making planned and unplanned role transitions. *Journal of Nursing Administration 27(9):17-23.*

Sape, G.P. (1985). Coping with comparable worth. *Harvard Business Review 63(3):145-152.*

Sands, J.K. (1991). Avoiding the pitfalls of job hunting. *Healthcare Trends &*

Transitions 3(1):52-55.

Sawyers, J. (1993). Defining your role in ambulatory care: Clinical nurse specialist or nurse practitioner? *Clinical Nurse Specialist 7(1):4-7.*

Shamansky, S. (1981). Marketing nurse practitioner services. *The Nurse Practitioner 6:42, 50-51.*

Soehren M.M., Schumann, L. (1994). Enhanced role opportunities available to the CNS/nurse practitioner. *Clinical Nurse Specialist 8(3):123-127.*

Styles, M.M. (1985). The uphill battle for comparable worth. *Nursing Outlook 33(3):128-137.*

Sullivan, J.A., Dachelet, C.Z., Sultz, H.A., Henry, O.M. & Carrol, H.D. (1978). Overcoming barriers to the employment and utilization of the nurse practitioner. *American Journal of Public Health 68:1097-1103.*

Turner, S. (1998). Transitioning yourself into the new health care business. *Orthopedic Nursing 17(2):30-32.*

Tyler, L. (1990). Watch out for "red flags" on a job interview. *Hospitals 64(14).*

Vogel, D. & Jackson, P. (1992). The interview. Reflections from the recruiter's side of the desk. *Healthcare Trends & Transitions 3(4):24-26.*

Walters, J.A. (1987). An innovative method of job interviewing. *The Journal of Nursing Administration 17(5):25-29.*

Winstead-Fry, P. (1990). *Career Planning: A Nurse's Guide to Career Advancement.* New York: National League for Nursing.

Wood, D. (1998). Effects of educational focus on a graduate nurse's initial choice of practice area. *Journal of Professional Nursing 14(4):214-219.*

CAREER-RELATED WEB SITES

U.S. Dept. of Labor, Bureau of Labor Statistics, economic data, section on regional data: **www.bls.gov**

Ability to send out resumes online to multiple employers listing positions. Can also develop job search criteria and be notified via e-mail when matching positions become available: **www.careerpath.com**

Information on impact of demographic data on the economy: **www.census.gov**

The Riley Guide, general career advice: **www.dbm.com/jobguide**

Career information specifically for nurses: **www.nursingspectrum.com**

10

Legal and Regulatory Aspects of Advanced Practice

Introduction

The first nurse registration statutes were passed in 1903 in New York, North Carolina, New Jersey, and Virginia. By 1923, all states had nurse registration acts on their books. In 1938, the second phase of such legislation began with New York's mandatory practice act which defined two levels of nurses: registered and practical (1).

Today, all state statutes relating to nursing contain a definition of nursing, requirements for licensure and for endorsing those licensed in other states, and rules and regulations governing the licensure processes and the board of examiners. The key to practice is the definition of nursing. This is especially important for nurses whose practice encroaches on what has traditionally been hallowed medical turf. In this chapter, we will examine some legal aspects of the roles, including state nurse practice acts, credentialing, prescriptive authority, reimbursement, and malpractice issues.

Nurse Practice Acts

In 1955, the American Nurses Association proposed a model definition of nursing for state nurse practice acts. In part, this definition reads: "The practice of professional nursing means the performance for compensation of any act in the observation, care, and counsel of the ill, injured, or infirm, or in the maintenance of health or prevention of illness of others . . .the foregoing shall not be deemed to include acts of diagnosis or prescription of therapeutic or corrective measures" (2).

Many states used this definition in their acts. In 1970, acknowledging advanced practice roles, the American Nurses Association suggested that states might wish to consider modifying their definitions if they appeared too restrictive. To that end, the following definition was proposed: "A professional nurse may also perform such additional acts, under emergency or other special conditions, which may include special training, as are recognized by the medical and nursing professions as proper to be performed by a professional nurse under such conditions, even though such acts might otherwise be considered diagnosis and prescription" (2). Clearly, this definition spells out the need for special preparation while at the same time recognizing the overlap with medicine that delivery of care by advanced practitioners may require. In 1971 Idaho became the first state to incorporate advanced practice into its definition of nursing (3).

A survey of state boards of nursing in 1980 revealed that 15 states retained a traditional definition of nursing similar or identical to the one proposed as a model in 1955 by ANA. Preparation for advanced practice roles had begun many decades earlier, but states have been slow to recognize advanced practice nurses in their practice acts. A few states led the way, however; for example, Idaho in 1971, Arizona in 1973, and Alabama and Rhode Island in 1982 (5, 8, 9, 10, 16).

Rhode Island's 1982 nurse practice act states, in part, that "The assessment of an individual's health status, identification of health care needs, determination of health care goals . . . and the development of a plan of nursing care to achieve these goals" are part of the role of the professional nurse (5). One of the earliest states to recognize advanced practice nurses in its nurse practice act, Rhode Island's regulations are quite liberal; there are no stipulations for physician supervision of nurse practitioners, clinical nurse specialists, or nurse anesthetists. Nurse-midwives have their own separate law and are not under the board of nursing (9).

The National Council of State Boards of Nursing published a new model nursing practice act in 1982. It's definition of practice is: "The `practice of nursing' means assisting individuals or groups to maintain or attain optimal health throughout the life process by assessing their health status, establishing a diagnosis, planning and implementing a strategy of care to accomplish defined goals, and evaluating responses to care and treatment" (6). This definition is important because it includes diagnosis and treatment under the purview of nursing.

Following these examples, nurses in other states began to examine their nurse practice acts to determine who holds regulatory control over advanced nursing practice. Alaskan nurses were successful more than a decade ago in updating their nurse practice act to include a definition of an advanced nurse practitioner, as well as regaining control over all levels of nursing (7). Other states followed in updating their practice acts to include nurse-midwives, nurse anesthetists, nurse practitioners, psychiatric clinical nurse specialists, and finally, all advanced practice nurses. In some states, nurse-midwives and nurse anesthetists have separate laws and may not be under the jurisdiction of the board of nursing.

By 1999, 43 states and the District of Columbia included advanced practice nurses in their nurse practice acts, with the boards of nursing as the sole authority on the scope of practice of these nurses. In 17 states and the District of Columbia, no requirements were included specifying physician collaboration or physician supervision of advanced practice nurses. Sixteen other states recognized advanced practice nurses in their nurse practice acts and had their board of nursing as the sole authority for the scope of practice, but required physician collaboration. In 9 states, the board of nursing has sole authority, but the scope of practice for nurse practitioners requires physician supervision. Five states recognized advanced practice nurses, but required authorization of the scope of practice by both boards of nursing and medicine. In 2 states, there was no title protection for advanced practice nurses and they functioned under a broad nurse practice act. Thirty-eight states and the District of Columbia recognized clinical nurse specialists within the advanced practice nurse category; for some of these, only psychiatric mental health clinical nurse specialists were so recognized.

Either under the umbrella "advanced practice nurse" or in separate legislation, by 1999 most states recognized nurse-midwives and nurse anesthetists. In a couple of states, there is no title protection for nurse-midwives and one need not be a nurse to be licensed as a midwife.

State legislation and the rules and regulations promulgated under legislation provides title protection (i.e., no one without the requisite credentials can use the title nurse practitioner, etc.), defines scope of practice, delineates any requirements for physician supervision or collaboration and for protocols, and may address hospital admitting and discharge privileges, as well as prescriptive authority and reimbursement (9, 73).

Educational qualifications vary widely among the 50 states and the District of Columbia. Some require master's preparation for one or more of the 4 advanced practice roles, some require only additional preparation appropriate to the role beyond basic nursing education, and some substitute national certification by an appropriate certifying body for specific educational credentials. A number of states are phasing in the requirements for a master's degree for all advanced practice nurses and may grandfather or grandmother in advanced practice nurses from certificate programs who have a bachelor's, an associate degree, or a diploma (9, 73).

One of the greatest barriers to practice for advanced practice nurses in the past has been legislative regulation (4, 8, 11, 16). In 23 states, as of 1999, at least some if not all advanced practice nurses could practice only with physician collaboration or supervision. In a study sponsored by the Bureau of Health Professions of the Health Resources and Services Administration, U.S. Public Health Service, investigators found wide variations among states in the practice environments for nurse practitioners and certified nurse-midwives (as well as for physician assistants). When practice environments are favorable, and these environments include statutory regulation, there is a greater supply of advanced practice nurses (11).

Recommendations for changing state statutory language are helpful to advanced practice nurses as they seek changes in states that do not allow full independent processes (12, 16). Research is also very helpful in influencing regulatory processes. Criteria for analyzing licensure laws are also helpful in this process. In order to do an analysis, it is first necessary to obtain an annotated copy of the nurse practice act from a law library or from one's state senator or representative. Copies from the board of nursing are usually not annotated. Rules and regulations (referred to as R & R) governing the practice of the advanced practice nurse are promulgated separately and are published in a state code of rules available in a law library, from the statehouse bookstore, or through the state board of nursing. In several states, the state nurses association has put together a book of all legislation pertinent to the practice of advanced practice nurses including copies of the rule and regulations. The American Nurses Association has a publication as well (77).

It is also helpful to examine the statutes for medicine and pharmacy. Criteria for this analysis include: attributing the usual meaning to terms used in the statutes and rules and regulations unless specified otherwise; examining the intent of the statutes and rules and regulations; examining and interpreting any amendments; and determining whether there is harmony or cacophony among the various statutes and rules and regulations governing or having an impact on the practice of advanced practice nurses (13).

Special Legislation for Expanded Nursing Practice

In addition to nurse practice acts and the rules and regulations guiding the practice of advanced practice nurses related to those acts, other pieces of legislation have direct bearing on the scope of practice of these nurses. Among the most important are laws governing who may have prescriptive authority and under what circumstances, and laws regarding direct third-party reimbursement for professional services.

Prescriptive Privileges

Until the 1938 Federal Food, Drug, and Cosmetic Act, consumers had access to all non-narcotic prescriptive drugs and it was not uncommon for nurses to work independently from physicians and make drug recommendations (8). Advanced practice nurses must surely have been among the nurses making recommendations or administering drugs, particularly nurse-midwives and nurse anesthetists, as well as public health nurses in many settings. After 1938, it took nearly three decades for advanced practice nurses to begin to reclaim this lost practice component. In 1975, North Carolina became the first state to grant prescriptive authority, limited though it was, to advanced practice nurses (8, 9). By 1999, advanced practice nurses in 10 states and the District of Columbia could prescribe drugs, including controlled substances, independent of physician supervision. In an additional 31 states, advanced practice nurses could prescribe drugs, including controlled substances, with some physician involvement. Nine states allowed advanced practice nurses to prescribe drugs, excluding controlled substances, with some physician involvement. Nurse practitioners have authority to dispense drug samples in 25 states. In states where this is not specifically permitted or prohibited by statute, it may have become the standard of practice (9, 74).

Clinical nurse specialists have prescriptive privileges in 32 states, although some privileges apply to psychiatric-mental health CNSs only. In 25 states, nurse anesthetists have prescriptive authority; in some states this means only authority to administer anesthetic agents and in others to prescribe beyond this function. Nurse-midwives can prescribe in 45 states. Mandated physician involvement varies (9, 73, 82).

Some state statutes are very limiting, and in some states only certain categories of advanced practice nurses have prescriptive authority (9). Rules and regulations can include requirements for continuing education; special courses and/or examinations; notification of the boards of nursing and medicine and sometimes pharmacy as to the practice sites; exclusionary formularies; evidence of practice as an advanced practice nurse for a specified length of time; restriction of geographic area or setting; and other restrictions (8, 9, 17, 73). In Massachusetts, for example, advanced practice nurses authorized for prescriptive authority under state law must include a copy of the protocol with physician colleagues in their applications for such authority. In a number of states, both the board of nursing and the board of medicine regulate prescriptive authority for advanced practice nurses. The board of pharmacy plays a role in development of the approved formulary in some states and even in the granting of such authority to advanced practice nurses (9, 73).

Advanced practice nurses who are eligible for prescriptive privileges have to apply for these privileges in each individual state; there is no reciprocity between states at present. Often the application process is tedious and complicated. Many states require a written collaboration agreement between the advanced practice nurse and supervising or collaborating physician to be filed as part of this application process (see Appendix F). Some limit the number of advanced practice nurses who can collaborate with or be supervised by one physician. Special prescription pads may be required for advanced practice nurses that include the collaborating physician's name, a place for the physician's signature or printed name, and sometimes other restrictive language. All of these are ways for medicine and sometimes pharmacy to control the practice of nurses (9, 17, 73).

Studies of the prescription writing practices of nurse practitioners have revealed that they make effective and appropriate use of such privileges. But a study of employer resistance to authorizing prescriptive authority for nurse practitioners found that employer resistance was a significant factor in the failure of advance practice nurses to exercise their prescriptive authority in their practice (19).

It has taken nearly 25 years for the Federal Drug Enforcement Agency (DEA) to allow advanced practice nurses prescriptive authority for controlled substances. When the Controlled Substances Act was passed by Congress in 1970, provisions were not made for advanced practice nurses. Undeterred, some advanced practice nurses applied for and received DEA numbers, until in 1990 the DEA began to question the right of these nurses to do so under existing rules (16). Over the intervening years, rules and regulations were modified to include advanced practice nurses in the system. But until 1993, considerable controversy existed over allowing such nurses to have their own DEA numbers; in many states, legislation restricted advanced practice nurses to having DEA numbers only through affiliations with physicians. A 1993 DEA ruling grants advanced practice nurses the right to apply for and have their own DEA numbers. The full text of the regulation is in the *Federal Register* for June 1, 1993, volume 58, pages 31171-31175, and can be obtained through libraries housing this publication (21). Prescriptive authority for controlled substances for advanced practice nurses is still restricted by the states, however (9, 40, 73).

Eligible advanced practice nurses, under the DEA ruling, can submit an application for a DEA number. On this application, they are required to include information about the extent of prescriptive authority in the state(s) in which they practice. The DEA has issued a guide for this process entitled *Mid-Level Practitioner's Manual.* Some states continue to misuse the DEA number, requiring it in order to recognize the authority of providers to prescribe. Under federal law, the DEA number is required only for prescription of controlled substances.

In some states, however, all prescription drugs are controlled substances, but are sorted into schedules of drugs as defined by the United States Food and Drug Administration, only some of which are protected under this DEA regulation. This adds to the confusion for all health care professionals and may limit access to care for patients (21, 55).

In the few states where prescriptive privileges are restrictive, many nurses in advanced practice are writing prescriptions on presigned pads, using collaboratively developed protocols, writing prescriptions and then having the physician sign them, distributing stock medications, calling in prescriptions to pharmacies, and/or writing prescriptions and signing the names of both the advanced practice nurse and the physician (8, 9).

In order for advanced practice nurses to attain full prescriptive authority in states that do not grant full independent practice, the first step is to analyze the existing nurse practice acts and the rules and regulations governing authorization to prescribe (72). After completing this background work, it is time to assess the political climate and lay the foundation for an amendment or a new bill to be filed. Legislators sympathetic to advanced practice nurses and their staff members can be extremely helpful in this process. Drawing together the organizations representing the different advanced practice nurses so that they can be perceived as speaking with one voice can be very useful. The experience of groups that already have prescriptive authority can be very instructive to this process. Typically, nurse anesthetists, nurse-midwives, and psychiatric mental health clinical specialists have led the way, particularly in more urban areas with high ratios of providers to population. In rural areas and those designated as medically underserved, nurse practitioners and nurse-midwives may have already fought for and won prescriptive privileges. In some states, nurse anesthetists have these privileges because they are considered inherent to their practice of administering anesthetic agents. The wording in the rules and regulations governing their practice could be helpful in drafting legislation (16, 55). Most important in the process is educating legislators and the public about the roles of advanced practice nurses. As Safriet noted, regulators have relied on physicians to define and describe what advanced practice nurses do or ought to be allowed to do (16).

Direct Third-Party Reimbursement

Direct third-party reimbursement for professional services is a second legislative issue with profound effects on the practice of advanced practice nurses. Details of the struggles of these nurses to be recognized by third-party payers are discussed in Chapter 8. Without adequate reimbursement schemes, advanced practice nurses cannot practice independently and are restricted in their practice roles and settings, and patients have limited access to the whole range of health care professionals (8, 16). Strategies similar to those suggested for attaining prescriptive authority can be employed to construct and pass legislation at the state level to provide direct reimbursement for advanced practice nurses (12, 13, 16, 56).

Second Licensure, Certification, or Authorization
In a number of states, second licensure, a certification process, or authorization by the board of nursing (and sometimes the board of medicine or the state education department) is used. Several states have a separate certified nurse-midwife board. Forty-four states require additional credentialing for nurse practitioners, 43 for nurse anesthetists and midwives, and 40 for clinical nurse specialists. In some states, all advanced practice nurses are credentialed under the board of nursing. In others, it varies, depending on the type of advanced practice nurse. Several states still do not formally credential clinical nurse specialists or only credential psychiatric mental health CNSs (9, 73). The rules and regulations for this credentialing vary considerably. Some states require only that advanced practice nurses apply for credentialing once they can meet the requirements (i.e., advanced educational preparation and/or national certification). The state then issues a second or a replacement license or other form of credentialing with the appropriate designation on it or a separate certificate with no change in the registered nurse license. For this process, some states require only a simple application and proof of graduation from an advanced practice program and/or national certification. Others require an extensive application procedure including transcripts, course syllabuses, preceptorships (sites, preceptors, number of hours) and program objectives. Several states require board of nursing approval of the professional certifying body in order for applicants to be eligible for advanced practice licenses (9, 73).

Designations for advanced practice nurses under state laws are as varied as the processes for attaining the titles. Certified nurse-midwife (CNM), certified registered nurse anesthetist (CRNA), nurse practitioner (NP), and clinical nurse specialist (CNS) are the most common but are not the only titles mandated in legislation. Some rules state that the advanced practice nurse is to use the designation of the national certifying body, for example, CNM from the American College of Nurse-Midwives certifying body, Registered Nurse Certified (RNC) for nurses certified by the National Certification Corporation (NCC), and RN,CS (registered nurse, certified specialist) for both clinical nurse specialists and nurse practitioners certified by the American Nurses Credentialing Center, a subsidiary of the American Nurses Association. To this, one might add the specialty: e.g., RN, CS-FNP. Several states spell out the designation the advanced practice nurse must use. For example, in New Hampshire and Nebraska nurse practitioners, nurse-midwives, and nurse anesthetists are ARNPs—advanced registered nurse practitioners. Advanced practice registered nurse (APRN), advanced practice nurse (APN), certified nurse practitioner (CNP), registered nurse practitioner (RNP), certified nurse specialist (CNS), certified registered nurse practitioner (CNRP) and certified registered nurse-midwife (CRNM) are other designations. Nurse practitioners may also use initials to indicate specialty: FNP (family nurse practitioner), GNP (geriatric nurse practitioner), and so on (9, 24).

While we are struggling with issues of credentialing of advanced practice nurses in the United States, our colleagues in Ontario, Canada, have experienced what even might be considered a paradigm shift in the way health care professionals are credentialed. At the end of 1993, the regulated Health Professions Act was passed. One intent of this legislation was to create consistency in the way in which health professions are regulated. All members of regulated professions, and this includes nursing, must be registered through their respective colleges; in the case of nurses, this would be the College of Nurses of Ontario. Each profession has a broad and general scope of practice statement describing what the profession does and the methods its members use, and protected titles, such as nurse, registered nurse, and registered practical nurse. Nurse practitioner is not among these titles at present. This legislation eliminates exclusive control by any profession of any of the 13 acts considered potentially harmful if performed by unqualified persons. For example putting an instrument, hand or finger beyond any body orifice or into an artificial opening in the body is such an act. Nurses are limited by regulation as to when they may perform such acts, but physicians are not (41, 70, 71). This is an interesting model to contemplate and may influence health care in this country. Advanced practice nurses in other Canadian provinces, Great Britain, Australia, Israel, and other countries are struggling with issues of credentialing (57-60).

It is clear that the creation of advanced practice roles for nurses has had an impact on how we choose, in a legal sense, to define nursing practice. It is equally clear that the roles have incited dissension about the scope of practice and control of practice, not only within the profession but with other health care providers, most notably physicians. If we are to retain, or in some cases regain, full control of our practice and how it is to be defined, we will have to become more active politically.

Certification and Credentialing

National Certification

In 1973, the American Nurses' Association announced its intention to initiate a pilot program for national certification to recognize excellence in nursing practice. The first 191 nurses were certified in 1974 and honored in a formal ceremony in January, 1975 (22).

In the ANA bylaws adopted at the 1976 convention, each practice division is charged with providing "recognition of professional achievement and excellence in its area of concern" (23). The original intention, which was to recognize excellence, yielded to pressures by consumers, third-party payers, and others, so that by 1978, the year in which ANA voted to fund the certification process for two years, the purposes had expanded. Dr. Mauksch, chairperson of the Interdivisional Council on Certification, identified these purposes as: assurance of quality beyond basic licensure; identification of nurses who may be directly reimbursable for services; and recognizing achievement and quality of practice (23).

Certification in 1978 included the following specialties: maternal-gynecological nursing; psychiatric/mental health nursing; clinical specialist in psychiatric and mental health nursing; adult and family nurse practitioners; community health nursing; gerontological nursing; pediatric nurse practitioner (ambulatory); clinical specialist in medical-surgical nursing; and medical-surgical nurse. By the end of that same year, 1,350 nurses had been certified. In 1979, school nurse-practitioner, nursing of acute and chronically ill children, and high-risk perinatal nursing were added (23).

The American Nurses Credentialing Center (ANCC), a subsidiary of the American Nurses Association, offers certification examinations for advanced practice nurses as both clinical nurse specialists and nurse practitioners and an advanced examination in nursing administration requiring a master's degree. Materials from ANCC include the educational guidelines for programs preparing advanced clinical nurse specialists certified by ANCC. These include adult psychiatric and mental health nursing, child and adolescent psychiatric and mental health nursing, medical-surgical nursing, gerontological nursing, community health nursing, and home health nursing. Pediatric, adult, acute care, school, family, and gerontological nurse practitioners are certified by ANCC.

As of 1999, 150,000 nurses held current ANCC certification as clinical nurse specialists, as nurse practitioners, and in nursing administration advanced level, as well as generalist certification in 12 specialty areas (baccalaureate degree required) (24). What these figures do not reveal is how many nurses hold dual certification in advanced practice roles: a study of ANCC certified nurses generated an estimate of 8% (27).

In 1980, by mutual consent with ANA, the Nurses' Association of the American College of Obstetricians and Gynecologists (now the Association of Women's Health, Obstetric, and Neonatal Nurses or AWHONN) took over the credentialing of obstetric/gynecologic nurse practitioners, inpatient obstetric nurses, and neonatal intensive care nurses. By 1993, this group changed its name to the National Certification Corporation for the Obstetric, Gynecologic, and Neonatal Nursing Specialties, and had added neonatal nurse practitioner, low risk neonatal nurse, high risk obstetric nurse, ambulatory women's health care nurse, and reproductive endocrinology/infertility nurse. Maternal newborn nurse was the added to NCC certification options, and in 1995 the title "obstetric/gynecologic nurse practitioner" was changed to "women's health care nurse practitioner" (25).

In 1997, NCC placed 3 examinations on hiatus: ambulatory women's health care, high-risk obstetrical nursing, and reproductive endocrinology/infertility nursing (26). In 1999, it added new subspecialty (modular) examinations for primary care nurse practitioners in obstetrics and gynecological reproductive health for nurse practitioners already certified by AANP, ACNM, ANCC or NCBPN-P. Also, NCC offers a breast feeding subspeciality examination and electronic fetal monitoring examination (25,61). By January of 2000, candidates for certification as neonatal nurse practitioners must have a master's degree (25).

As of 1999, the National Certification Corporation had certified the following numbers of advanced practice nurses: 9,327 women's health nurse practitioners and 2,650 neonatal nurse practitioners (25). The American Nurses Association through the American Nurses Credentialing Center continues to certify those groups listed for 1978 and 1979 with the exception of maternal/newborn nurses, and now requires a master's degree for its nurse practitioner, clinical nurse specialist, and nursing administration advanced certification programs (24).

Occupational health is a new component of community health. The American Board for Occupational Health Nurses certifies nurses for this area of practice. The American College of Nurse-Midwives (ACNM) Certification Council continues to certify nurse-midwives who are graduates of the programs which it accredits. As of the end of 1998, the American College of Nurse-Midwives listed 7,000 certified nurse-midwives (10). The Council on Certification of Nurse Anesthetists certifies nurse anesthetists in a manner similar to that of the ACNM through its Council on Certification. Of the nearly 27,000 nurse anesthetists in the U.S., virtually all are certified, since certification is required to practice (68). The National Association of Pediatric Nurse Associates and Practitioners (NAPNAP) sponsors, through its National Certification Board of Pediatric Nurse Practitioners and Nurses (NCEPNP), the National Qualifying Examinations for Pediatric Nurse Practitioners. Since 1977, this group has certified several thousand pediatric nurse practitioners. More than two dozen additional nursing organizations and several interdisciplinary associations are now involved in credentialing nurses. Seven of these certify advanced practice nurses (30). (See Appendix B.)

In 1994, the American Academy of Nurse Practitioners began to offer national certification through examination for adult and family nurse practitioners. Candidates have to be graduates of approved master's programs or petition the Certification Board for other credentials they believe entitle them to sit for the examination (69). Several specialty organizations offer certification and some of these include advanced practice roles. The Oncology Nursing Certification Corporation (the certifying body for the Oncology Nursing Society) (28) and the American Association of Critical Care Nurses are two examples of specialty organizations that offer certification examinations for an advanced level of practice (63). Other nursing organizations offer certification examinations for specialty practice, but not necessarily at an advanced practice level in one of the four advanced practice nursing roles.

Several important and troubling questions are raised by the plethora of credentialing bodies and examinations. Credentialing does not have a uniform meaning, and the criteria for certification and recertification vary (29). Educational requirements to sit for a certification examination range from holding a license to practice as an RN to a minimum of a master's degree for some advanced practice certification (30). The cost of certification to the candidate is considerable, and achievement of certification sometimes goes unrecognized by the employer.

In 1996, the Oncology Nursing Certification Corporation hosted a state-of-the-knowledge conference on nursing certification with representatives from 24 specialty certification organizations. The consensus among attendees was that only specialty organizations have the knowledge to develop standards and credentialing for specialty practice and that nurses who are certified need to communicate the meaning of this credentialing to health care providers and the public (31).

Recertification is a second important issue related to certification as credentialing. The existing national certifying bodies have a variety of means of maintaining certification including retesting, demonstrating continuation in practice, and mandatory continuing education. Critics have argued that mandatory continuing education, the most common mechanism for recertification, does not necessarily reflect the professional development needs nor assure continuing competency (29, 31).

Uncertainty Regarding Certification and Credentialing Issues
In late 1994, the American Association of Colleges of Nursing issued a position statement on certification and regulation of advanced practice nurses. In that statement, members of the association (deans and chairpersons of colleges, schools, and departments of nursing in college and university settings) urged that advanced practice should mean graduate preparation and that certifying bodies should meet national standards to be developed and implemented by some separate body such as the American Board of Nursing Specialties (ABNS) (67). This organization, founded in 1991 with 8 charter organizations, resulted from the inability of the American Nurses Association, the National Federation of Specialty Nursing Organizations (NFSNO, founded in 1973), and other specialty groups to reach consensus on criteria for credentialing. A number of these organizations were unwilling to require a minimum of a baccalaureate degree for any certification examination and are therefore not recognized by

ABNS (31).

Another question raised by issues of certification and the broader topic of credentialing, discussed earlier in this chapter, is what nurses are to be called who are credentialed beyond the basic nursing preparation that allowed them to sit for licensure and use the initials RN.

Titling is a troublesome issue, as it involves not only professional but also public recognition of who nurses are and what differentiates who we are and how we practice; that is, what we are allowed to do under nurse practice acts and what the public has a right to expect from us. In her landmark work on specialization in nursing, Styles (32) urged us as a profession to empower ourselves through self-regulation. The new millennium promises to urge us forward as the nation struggles with chaos in health care and the place of advanced practice nurses in managed care, care systems, and other emerging models for care delivery and funding.

The issues of certification and credentialing for advanced practice roles are not likely to be resolved quickly. They are critical issues for control of practice for advanced practice nurses, however. As has been pointed out, there are many fingers in the pie and the number appears to be growing. In addition to the National League for Nursing, the current accrediting body for schools of nursing, the American Association of Colleges of Nursing (AACN) has issued its position paper on the credentialing of advanced practice nurses (67), the National Council of State Boards of Nursing is considering issues of multistate licensure for advanced practice nurses (30, 62, 65, 75, 76), and the National Task Force on Quality Nurse Practitioner Education under the aegis of the National Organization of Nurse Practitioner Faculties (NONPF) has issued guidelines for the preparation of nurse practitioners (33). State approval of baccalaureate programs is necessary for graduates to it for NCLEX examinations and, if multistate licensure for advanced practice nurses comes to pass, might not schools also have to be approved so that their master's graduates are eligible for such licensure? Schools with nurse-midwifery and nurse anesthetist programs are accredited by the appropriate accrediting arm of their professional organizations in addition to the National League for Nursing (NLN) accreditation. In 1998, NLN adopted criteria developed by the National Task Force on Quality Nurse Practitioner Education (33). It remains for the future to determine what the role of the evolving Commission on Collegiate Nursing (CCNE) of AACN will be (30). Specialty organizations set the standards for practice and, in many cases, standards for educational preparation for advanced practice nurses which schools must meet in order for their graduates to be eligible to sit for the appropriate certification examination.

Pending National Legislation

Trends on a national level include moves by states to tighten licensing laws, increase professional accountability, require a master's degree for advanced practice roles, set national practice standards, use national certification as a credentialing mechanism, have stronger licensure laws and boards, put consumers on boards, develop equivalency examinations for educational programs and occupations, and put in place mechanisms to insure provider mobility as well as increased accountability, including multistate licensure.

In 1998, the National Council of State Boards of Nursing approved the final version of a document entitled a Mutual Recognition Model for Multistate Regulation of Nursing (MSR). As a consequence of the mobility of the population of the United States and the advent of the computer age and telehealth, those responsible for licensing health care professionals realized that continuing on the current path of licensure and other credentialing on a state-by-state basis raised some knotty legal questions as well as perpetuating what has become a cumbersome system. Adopting the MSR will permit registered nurses to practice (electronic or physical) across state lines without additional credentialing, as long as they hold one license to practice in their states of residency and are not under discipline or an agreement that restricts such practice (62, 65, 66, 75, 76).

As the 50 states contemplate signing on for MSR, the discussion continues about what to do with advanced practice nurses. Although uniform examination for entry level licensure in nursing has been in place for decades and licensure requirements are essentially identical, this is not the case at the advanced practice level (62, 65, 66, 75). The NCSBN has adopted in principle the concept of multistate licensure for advanced practice nurses, but, recognizing how complex this will be to accomplish, has set a different timeline. A task force comprised of representatives of NCSBN and of nurse practitioner, clinical nurse specialist, nurse-midwifery, and nurse anesthetist organizations has been meeting to address multistate licensure for advanced practice registered nurses (62, 65, 66, 75).

Issues of Legal Liability and Malpractice for Nurses in Advanced Practice

In this age of litigation, it is not surprising that nurses are concerned about their legal status and vulnerability. Nurses in advanced practice (and all registered nurses) can be and are being sued. However, after 18 months of data collection by the National Practitioner Data Bank (September 1990-February 1992), there is encouraging news. The rate of malpractice payments for nurses in advanced practice (per 1,000 practitioners) was 6.7 for nurse anesthetists, 5.5 for nurse-midwives, 1.0 for nurse practitioners, and 0.2 for registered nurses. (42). These figures compared with a rate of 32.2 for allopathic physicians. For the period 1990 through March of 1997, this same data bank reported that of 290 nursing medication errors, 11 involved advanced practice nurses (78).

In an examination of data from the National Practitioner Data Bank from the previous 18 months to July of 1993, only 2.4% of payments reported for malpractice were for nurses. Among these, 126 were for nurse anesthetists, 23 for nurse-midwives, and 14 for nurse practitioners. Birkholz points out that there may be under-reporting of payments because many advanced practice nurses are employees and the National Practitioner Data Bank does not require that either health care agencies or individual practitioner employees be named in reporting data (34). Claims are also several years old, because there is considerable lag time between filing a claim and settlement resulting in a payment (34).

The journal *Nurse Practitioner* has collected data on malpractice issues from its readers. In the most recent survey, 1,610 readers responded. Only 25 (0.016%) reported having had a claim against them. (The number of claims was 29.) Most of these occurred in the first 5 years of practice. To date, only 11 of the 29 claims had been settled. The cases are detailed in the report and are instructive for all nurses in advanced practice (35).

Issues for malpractice suits usually rest on what is reasonably prudent for a practitioner to do whose background is similar to that of the individual being sued. Malpractice means "the commission or omission of an act that harms a patient" (79, p. 24). Three questions follow: "What is the nature of the act that is of concern? . . . What are the qualifications of the nurse practitioner who performed the act? . . . Where was the care provided?" (80, pp. 34-35). Some specific questions are raised in the case of nurses in advanced practice. Who will the expert witness be—a nurse or a physician? By whom are policies and practices written? Does the literature reflect well-researched practice? Are the professional standards (see Appendix) for practice (ANA, AWHONN, NAPNAP, AACN, ONS, ACN, AANA and others) unrealistic ideals or are they attainable? What will be the standard of care for advanced practice? Some important questions have been raised about the legal dangers of written protocols and standards. If the standards are unreasonable, they may make the practitioner vulnerable (43).

Standards or guidelines for practice may come from a professional organization and then be translated into everyday practice through the development of protocols. The term "guidelines" is replacing "standards" as the preferred term for describing overall goals for practice, as it is less suggestive of rigid goals to be met for every patient. Protocols are commonly descriptions of the steps in care for specific conditions and/or presenting symptoms: assessment, diagnosis, intervention, follow-up, and evaluation of care.

Proponents of clinical practice guidelines point out that practitioners can reduce their risk of liability through identification of areas where there is a lack of consensus or where scientific evidence does not support current practices (36). Part of professional responsibility in relation to practice guidelines and protocols is to know the rules and regulations governing advanced practice under the state nurse practice act. The practice act may specify the scope of practice of an advanced practice nurse under the scope and standards of care defined by the specialty for which she/he is prepared by advanced education. In many states, protocols are mandatory, particularly for the practice of nurse practitioners, but may also be mandated for other advanced practice nurses. Sometimes the rules and regulations specify that the protocols be developed with or at least approved by the supervising or collaborating physician and even that they be filed with the boards of nursing and/or medicine. What these rules and regulations mean for legal liability for practice is that advanced practice nurses have the most protection under the law if they are practicing within the limits of the state nurse practice act.

An issue that relates, but is not the same as protocols, is the responsibility of the advanced practice nurse for follow-up of patients. Clinicians are required to make every reasonable attempt to follow-up with patients and have as much responsibility to do so as do the patients. State nurse practice acts may even have language requiring a nurse to act or intervene on behalf of a patient. The best protection a clinician can have is to ask of a situation: is follow-up required or justified; could the problem be threatening to the patient's health or life; and could serious harm result if the patient is not notified of the problem. Protocols might include follow-up such as for laboratory results, care for an abnormal Papanicolaou smear, and a return visit for test of cure following antibiotic therapy. Documenting the plan and then attempts to follow up in the patient's record will be important data. Computers are useful to set up tracking systems for laboratory tests and other data needing follow-up. In the absence of computers, log books are more than adequate as long as they are kept carefully (37).

The importance of documentation is not confined to follow-up. In the study of *Nurse Practitioner* readers, respondents who had been named in malpractice cases emphasized the importance of careful documentation and the use of language that might imply interventions beyond the scope of practice of the advanced practice nurse, such as counseling if one is not a counselor such as a psychiatric mental health clinical nurse specialist (35).

Related to documentation is the responsibility to be able to recall patients should a drug or device require such recall (38). Such recalls might include implants, drugs, and external medical devices. Patients' rights and informed consent are also critical issues and relate, in part, to drugs and devices that might be prescribed as well as all aspects of diagnosis and treatment (44, 45).

The rules and regulations promulgated for Medicare and Medicaid reimbursement legislation, as well as the Stark law addressing referrals among health care providers are so complex that "nurse practitioners and other primary care providers really need attorneys they can call for advice on a day-to-day basis" (81, p. 1). Some practices and agencies are even creating Medicare compliance programs with the help of attorneys (81). This is a new area of legal liability for advanced practice nurses.

Insurance Policies

As nurses become more vulnerable to suits, protection is important. Nurses choosing to protect their practices with malpractice insurance need to familiarize themselves with the risks covered in their policy, the amount of coverage provided, and the conditions spelled out (40, 46, 47).

It is important to understand the difference between an occurrence-based professional liability insurance policy and a claims-made policy. An occurrence-based policy provides coverage for any incident which *occurred* during the time the policy was in effect. A claims-made policy covers the nurse for any suit *filed* while the policy is in effect (40, 48, 80, 81).

Nurses should consider individual insurance policies even if they are covered by blanket institutional policies. Respondents to the *Nurse Practitioner* reader survey suggested careful consideration of the "practice impact of carrying malpractice insurance," and assertiveness on the part of the advanced practice nurse in demanding that an insurer pay for lawyers and defend the case (35, p. 30). It is important to explore all sources of policies. Group policies available through professional organizations may be cheaper, but it is important to scrutinize the coverage and compare carefully. State insurance laws will guide you as to who is issuing professional liability policies.

Be sure to check whether a policy will cover your practice as a nurse practitioner, clinical nurse specialist, nurse-midwife, or nurse anesthetist whatever your setting and mode of practice. Does the policy cover all your professional activities? Does it duplicate other insurance you may have? What are the exclusions? Are they important to your practice? What are the premiums? Remember, these are tax deductible as a professional expense. Will the policy pay a reasonable amount? Is there a limit on the amount per incident or on total coverage? If so, is it adequate? How is payment made for a claim? Does it cover legal fees? Can claims be settled without your consent? Must the claim be determined to be valid before a legal defense can begin? What are your responsibilities as the insured party? (40, 49). Given the malpractice insurance crisis for advanced practice of the 1980s, nurses must be well informed and should participate in legislative activity regarding malpractice insurance (50). Furthermore, they must assist in providing accurate data concerning liability claims (35, 51, 52).

In 1978, Senator Daniel K. Inouye of Hawaii first introduced a bill to establish a no-fault federal malpractice compensation system. Health care professionals could subscribe. The intent was to curb the destructive forces present in the suit-conscious private enterprise system that pit providers and consumers against each other in the legal arena (53). To date, no such bill has been passed. This attempt, however, represents an important effort to call off the accelerating legal cold war between health care professionals and the patients they serve. Perhaps such a plan will finally come to fruition under managed care or through the creation of care systems.

It is obvious that, if present trends continue, more and

more persons will choose professions with fewer legal risks, even though the monetary rewards may be less. The cost of malpractice insurance for some medical specialties already dissuades many. Where the spiraling of the legal costs of health care will take us is not clear. What is evident is that the present obsession with malpractice litigation encourages defensive practice on the part of the professions, increases costs for patients and/or third-party reimbursement programs, and undermines the fundamental trust relationship inherent in the caring professions.

Summary

The nurse in advanced practice needs to know about the legal and regulatory aspects of her or his role. This includes knowing the legal definitions for practice, including state nurse practice acts and state and federal legislation affecting practice, being aware of the standards and scope of practice as defined by professional organizations and what these mean from a legal perspective for advanced practice, and paying attention to documents such as the Code for Nurses and the Patient's Bill of Rights. The nurse who can speak with authority about the role and what responsibilities it encompasses is in an optimal position to define that role. If she or he is unable to be articulate about what constitutes the advanced practice role, others may dictate what that role is to be (54).

REFERENCES

1. Bullough, B. (1976). Influences on role expansion. *American Journal of Nursing 76:1476-1481.*
2. Kelly, L.Y. (1974). Nursing practice acts. *American Journal of Nursing 74:1310-1319.*
3. Bellocq, J.A. (1988). Part I: Florida's nurse practitioner act — defining practice. *Florida Nursing Review 2(3):3.*
4. Safriet, B.J. (1998). Still spending dollars, still searching for sense: Advanced

practice nursing in a era of regulatory and economic turmoil. *Advanced Practice Nursing Quarterly 4(3):24-33.*
5. Carroby, J.J. (Nov. 15, 1982). Governor's letter to health care professionals. State of Rhode Island and Providence Plantations, Executive Chamber.
6. The Model Nursing Practice Act. (1982). Chicago: The National Council of State of State Broads of Nursing, Inc.
7. Bertholf, C.B. (1986). Alaska implements new prescription regulations for advanced NPs. *The Nurse Practitioner 11(4):10, 15-16.*
8. Inglis, A.D. & Kjervik, D.K. (1993). Empowerment of advanced practice nurses: Regulation reform needed to increase access to care. *Journal of Law, Medicine, and Ethics 21:193-205.*
9. Pearson, L.J. (1999). Annual update of how each state stands on legislative issues affecting advanced nursing practice. *Nurse Practitioner 24(1):16-83.*
10. American College of Nurse Midwives, Washington, D.C.
11. Sercenski, E.S., Sansom, S., Bazell, C., Salmon, M.E. & Mullan, F. (1994). State practice environments and the supply of physician assistants, nurse practitioners, and certified nurse-midwives. *The New England Journal of Medicine 331:1266-1271.*
12. Birkholz, G. & Walker, D. (1994). Strategies for state statutory language changes granting fully independent nurse practitioner practice. *Nurse Practitioner 19(1):54-58.*
13. Hall, J.K. (1994). How to analyze nurse practitioner licensure laws. *Nurse Practitioner 18(8):31-34.*
14. Mahoney, D.F.(1992). Nurse practitioners as prescribers: Past research trends and future study needs. *The Nurse Practitioner 17(1):44; 47-48; 50-51.*
15. Harkless, G.E.(1989). Prescriptive authority: Debunking common assumptions. *The Nurse Practitioner 14(8),57-58; 60-61.*
16. Safriet, B.J. (1992). Health care dollars and regulatory sense. *Yale Journal on Regulation 9:417-488.*
17. Gunn, I.P., Tobin, M.H., Rupp, R.M. & Blumenreich, G.A. (1990). Nurses and prescriptive authority. *Specialty Nursing Forum 2(1): 1, 3-6.*
18. Pew Health Professions Commission. (1994). *Primary Care Workforce 2000.* San Francisco: University of California.
19. Mahoney, D.F. (1995). Employer resistance to state authorized prescriptive authority for NPs. *Nurse Practitioner 20(1):58-61.*
20. Mittelstadt, P. (1991). New rules expand role of NPs, CNSs. *The American Nurse 23(10):10.*
21. Havens, D.M..H. & Zink, R.L. (1993). Nurses achieve victory on prescriptive authority at DEA. *Journal of Pediatric Health Care 7:234-237.*
22. National certification. An idea that's here for good. (1981). *The American Nurse 13:11.*

23. ANA funds certification program for two years. New areas added. (1978). *American Journal of Nursing 78:534-541.*

24. American Nurses Credentialing Center 1999 Board Certification Catalog. (1999). Washington, DC: American Nurses Credentialing Center.

25. *NCC News.* (1999: Spring, Summer). Chicago: The National Certification Corporation.

26. *NCC News.* (1998: Fall). Chicago: The National Certification Corporation.

27. American Nurses Credentialing Center. (1995). Certified nurse demographic survey. *Credentialing News, Fall/Winter, 1994-1995.*

28. Oncology Nursing Certification Corporation. (1995). *Test Bulletin.*

29. Knapp, J.E. (1990). Continuing competency: A search for clarification. *Specialty Nursing Forum 3(2):1; 6-7.*

30. Hodnicki, D.R. (1998). Advanced practice nursing certification: Where do we go from here? *Advanced Practice Nursing Quarterly 4(3):34-43.*

31. ONCC Research Committee and Executive Staff. (1999). Report of the state-of-the-knowledge conference on U.S. nursing certification. *Image 21(1):51-55.*

32. Styles, M.M. (1989). *On Specialization in Nursing: Toward a New Empowerment.* Kansas City, MO: American Nurses Foundation.

33. National Task Force on Quality Nurse Practitioner Education (1997). Criteria for Evaluation of Nurse Practitioner Programs. Washington, DC: National Organization for Nurse Practitioner Faculties.

34. Birkholz, G. (1995). Malpractice data from the national practitioner data bank. *Nurse Practitioner 20(3):32-35.*

35. Pearson, L. & Birkholz, G. (1995). Report on the 1994 readership survey on NP experiences with malpractice issues. *Nurse Practitioner 20(3):18, 21-22, 24-26, 29-30.*

36. Jacox, A. (1993). Addressing variations in nursing practice/technology through clinical practice guidelines methods. *Nursing Economic$ 11:170-172.*

37. Stock, C. (1993). Follow-up: How much is enough? *Contemporary Ob/Gyn-NP 1(4):19-20.*

38. Henry, P.F. (1994). Duty to recall—the NPs role. *Nurse Practitioner Forum 5(2):62.*

39. Mastrangelo, R. (1993). Are you covered? Make sure your liability insurance is up to par. *Advance for Nurse Practitioners 1(5):15-20.*

40. Peters, S. (1999). Completing the 'right to write' controlled substance prescribing. *Advance for Nurse Practitioner 7(1):59-61.*

41. Risk, M. (1994 October). Protecting the title "nurse practitioner"—a regulatory dilemma. *College Communique, 5.*

42. The NPDB sums up months of malpractice experience. (1992). *American Journal of Nursing 92:9.*

43. Moniz, D.M. (1992). The legal danger of written protocols and standards of practice. *Nurse Practitioner 17(9):58-60.*

44. Koniak-Griffin, D. (1987). Challenges for the clinical nurse specialist in the

legal arena. *Clinical Nurse Specialist 1(3):142-147.*4

45. Moss, K.F. (1985). California supreme court defines standard of care for NPs. *The Nurse Practitioner 10(5):39-40, 42.*

46. Trandel-Korenchuk, D.M. & Trandel-Korenchuk, K.M. (1979). Nursing malpractice insurance: A review of one policy. *The Nurse Practitioner 4:11, 13, 15, 16-17, 19.*

47. Cotterell, Mitchell & Fifer, Inc. (1993). *Advantage, Spring issue, 5-8.*

48. Crane, M. (1979). Professional liability insurance: Occurrence versus claims-made policies. *Newsletter of the Council of Primary Health Care Nurse Practitioners 2:6.*

49. Brooke, P.S. (1989). The legal side: Shopping for liability insurance. *American Journal of Nursing 89(2):171-172.*

50. Northrup, C.E. (1980). Responding to the malpractice crisis. *American Journal of Nursing 80:2245-2246.*

51. Pearson, L.J. (1987). Comprehensive actuarial data on nurse practitioners . . . at long last. *The Nurse Practitioner 12(12):6, 9-10.*

52. Pearson, L.J. (1987). The liability insurance crisis. *The Nurse Practitioner 12(6):8-10.*

53. Senator Inouye introduces bill to set up no-fault federal malpractice system. (1978). *American Journal of Nursing 78:187, 208.*

54. Klein, C.A. (1986). Scope of practice. The Nurse Practitioner 11(11): 67, 71-72.

55. Minarik, P.A. (1993). Legislative and regulatory update: DEA registration for midlevel practitioners. *Clinical Nurse Specialist 7:319-329.*

56. Henry, P.F. (1994). Seeking legal authority to prescribe. *Nurse Practitioner Forum 5:203-204.*

57. Stilwell, B.(1984). The nurse in practice. *Nursing Mirror 158:17-22.*

58. Chiarella, M. (1998). Independent, autonomous, or equal: What do we really want? *Clinical Excellence for Nurse Practitioners 2:293-299.*

59. Shvarts, S. & Frenkel, D.A. (1998). Nurses in Israel: The struggle for regulating the profession. *Clinical Excellence for Nurse Practitioners 2:376-382.*

60. Muxlow, J. (1999, 1 Aug.). Advanced practice nurses in Nova Scotia. Personal communication.

61. NCC expands and revises certain examinations. (1999, June). *Nurse Practitioner World News, 21.*

62. Multistate licensure and APRSs. (1999). *Nurse Practitioner World News 4(2):22.*

63. Hravnak, M., Rosenzweig, M.Q., Rust, D. & Magdic, K. (1998). Scope of practice, credentialing, and privileging. In: R.M. Kleinpell & M.R. Piano (Eds.). *Practice Issues for the Acute Care Nurse Practitioner* (pp. 41-66). New York: Springer.

64. Nicholas, P. (1995). Issues in certification versus advanced practice licensure. *Nurse Practitioner 20(3):12.*

65. Chaffee, M. (1998). Changes proposed for RN licenses. *Nursing Economic$*

16(1):45-47.
66. Sharp, N. (1998). The drama of a paradigm shift: Looking at APRN licensure after the year 2000. *Nurse Practitioner 23(6):142-143*.
67. American Association of Colleges of Nursing. (1994). Certification and regulation of advanced practice nurses. Position Statement. Washington, DC: American Association of Colleges of Nursing.
68. Waugaman, W.R. & Foster, S.D. (1995). CRNAs: an enviable legacy of patient service. *Advanced Practice Nursing Quarterly 1(1):21-28*.
69. American Academy of Nurse Practitioners. (1994). *National Competency-based Certification Examinations for Adult and Family Nurse Practitioners*. Booklet on certification examinations.
70. Risk, M. (1994 March). RHPA: Innovative, exciting and complex. *College Communique 3, 8-13, 28-29*.
71. Scope of practice and controlled acts model. (1994 March). *College Communique, 99-93*.
72. Hamrie, A.B. (1998). Using research to influence the regulatory process. *Advanced Practice Nursing Quarterly 4(3):44-50*.
73. Minarik, P.A. & Tyner, I. (1999). Update on clinical nurse specialist recognition and prescriptive authority. *Clinical Nurse Specialist 13(3):140-144*.
74. Wiltz, P., Zimmer, P.A, & Scarcliff, K.J. (1999). NP authority to request, receive, and/or dispense drug samples: A state-by-state study. *Nurse Practitioner World News 4(1):3-4, 18-22*.
75. Stock, C.M. (1997). Practicing nursing across state lines: Changing times require changing nursing regulations. *Contemporary Nurse Practitioner 2(4):27-28*.
76. Peters, S. (1998). Multistate licensure. *Advance for Nurse Practitioners, 6(5):63-64, 84*.
77. American Nurses Association. (1999). *1999 Nursing Licensure Guidelines*. Washington, DC: American Nurses Publishing.
78. Carson, W.Y. (1999). Legal issues and advanced practice. In: M.D. Mezey & D.O. McGivern. *Nurses, Nurse Practitioners* (3rd ed., pp. 394-421). New York: Springer.
79. Morrison, C.A. (1999). Evolving legal trends affect NPs. *Advance for Nurse Practitioners 7(5):24*.
80. Hravnak, M., Rosenzweig, M.Q., Rust, D., & Magdie, K. (1998). Reimbursement, liability, and insurance. In: R.M. Kleinpell & M.R. Piano (Eds.). *Practice Issues for the Acute Care Nurse Practitioner*, (pp. 22-40). New York: Springer.
81. Buppert, Co. (1999). When NPs need attorneys. *Nurse Practitioner World News 4(3):1, 15*.
82. Prescribing victory in Kansas. (1999: July, August). *The American Nurse, 7*.

BIBLIOGRAPHY

Blanchfield, K.C., Schwarzentraub, L. & Reisinger P.B. (1998). Development of telephone nursing practice standards. *Nursing Economic$ 15(5):* 265-267.

Borchers, L. & Kee, C.C. (1999). An experience in telenursing. *Clinical Nurse Specialist 13:115-118.*

Bosma, J. (1997). Using nurse practitioner certification for state nursing regulations: An update. *Nurse Practitioner 22:213-216.*

Buppert, C. (1999). *Nurse Practitioner's Business Practice & Legal Guide.* Baltimore, MD: Aspen.

Buppert, C. (1999). PA/NP prescriber language on OTC drug labeling rejected. *Clinician News 3(6):14.*

Forward, D.C. (1998). Managing malpractice insurance. *American Journal of Nurs ing 98(3):16BB-16LL.*

Grant, M., Kinzie, A. & Landers, T. (1999). Writing prescriptions for family. *Advance for Nurse Practitioners 7(3):24.*

Hales, A., Karshmer, J., Montes-Sandoval, L. & Fiszbein, A. (1998). Preparing for prescriptive privileges: A CNS-physician collaborative model. Expanding the scope of the psychiatric-mental health clinical nurse specialist. *Clinical Nurse Specialist 12(2):73-80.*

Kleinpell, R.M. & Hayden, J. (1999). Longitudinal survey of acute care nurse practitioners. *Nurse Practitioner 24(8):105-106.*

Minarik, P.A. (1997). State legislative and regulatory forum. *Clinical Nurse Specialist 11(5):231.*

Nejedly, M.P., Broden, K., Knox, S.C., Jennings, A.F., et al. (1999). Prescribing guidelines based on a flexible scope of practice. *Clinical Excellence for Nurse Practitioners 3(2):73-79.*

Rustia, J.G. & Bartek, J.K. (1997). Managed care credentialing of advanced practice nurses. *Nurse Practitioner 22:90, 92, 99-100, 102-103.*

Sharp, N. (1997). Regional or multistate licensure: Is it coming soon? *Nurse Practitioner 22:170, 172-173.*

ONLINE RESOURCES

American Academy of Nurse Practitioners: **www.aanp.org**
American Association of Colleges of Nursing: **www.aacn.nche.edu**
American Association of Nurse Anesthetists Council on Certification of Nurse Anesthetists: **http://www.aana.com/proinfo/history.htm**
American College of Nurse Midwives Certification Council: **acnm.org**
American Nurses Credentialing Center: **www.nursingworld.org**

National Certification Board of Pediatric Nurse Practitioners and Nurses:
   info@pnpcert.org; website: **www.pnpcert.org**
National Certification Corporation for the Obstetric, Gynecologic, and
   Neonatal Nursing Specialties.
   For registration catalogue, certification maintenance:
                    www.nccnet.org/apps.html
   For studying for NCC examinations:
                    www.nccnet.org/certprep.htm
   To submit a change of address or name:
                    www.nccnet.org/contact.htm
National Council of State Boards of Nursing: **http://www.ncsbn.org**
National League for Nursing: **http://204.19.14/nlnac/criteria.htm**
National Organization of Nurse Practitioner Faculties:
   nonpf@aacn.nche.edu

11

Continuous Quality Improvement

Introduction

Since the passage of the Professional Standards Review Organization bill (PSRO-P.L.92-603) in 1972 and the ever-increasing involvement of third-party payers in monitoring the costs and quality of care, all health care providers have to concern themselves with some sort of evaluation and review system. The public is becoming increasingly vociferous in demanding accountability (1). Patients, employers, third parties, and other care systems are demanding that nurses be accountable for the cost and quality of the services they provide. Quality improvement represents a mechanism for accountability. In addition, a continuous quality improvement program can be structured to provide us with data to strengthen our case for direct third-party reimbursement, to demonstrate the unique contribution nurses can make to quality health care, and to document our acceptance by patients (1a, 1b).

Continuous Quality Improvement:
Some Definitions and Components

The focal point of health care quality has been quality assurance (QA). This notion of quality has expanded beyond the concepts of measuring, monitoring, and evaluation to include the manager's responsibility and initiatives for system quality (Total Quality Management). The key aspects of TQM, stemming from the works of Juran and Deming, are patient-orientation, commitment to quality by all levels and types of staff, organizational support and continuous improvement of the system as evidenced by prevention of problems and systematic, creative problem solving (3). Continuous quality improvement transcends the notion of QA as periodic evaluation of performance, as a reflection of quality, to become an integral part of the organization's vision which is operationalized in all facets of care delivery (3).

Attempts to define quality show the complexity of the concept. Any definition will reflect the biases of its author. At the same time, it is apparent that a quality improvement program must achieve at least a working agreement as to the quality of nursing care desired and must list the criteria that represent quality. One of the most useful definitions in the nursing literature states that quality of care is the observable characteristics that depict a desired and valued degree of excellence and its expected and observed variation (2).

Quality improvement (QI) programs are directed toward assuring some degree of excellence as defined by those responsible for the program and toward assuring accountability by health care providers for the quality of care they provide. An assumption in quality improvement is that every process can be improved. Juran (4) defines QI as "The organized creation of beneficial change . . . the attainment of unprecedented levels of performance."

The consumer should be the individual for whom we are assuring quality and to whom we are accountable. There are many, however, who would take issue with the consumer's rights or even ability to judge quality of care. Peers, institutions, and agencies, and increasingly managed care systems as well as credentialing, licensing, and accrediting bodies now usurp this prerogative (5).

Strategies to assure quality are many and varied. We have become familiar with words like peer review, audit, and chart or record review. It is possible to incorporate a number of these strategies into the quality improvement process.

Quality improvement programs have addressed one or more of three domains: structure, process, and outcome. *Structure evaluation* involves looking at how the setting, the conditions, and the environmental factors affect the quality of care. *Process evaluation* examines the activities and behaviors of the nurse. *Outcome* measures demonstrate changes in the behaviors and attitudes of the

patients.
The last component of quality improvement consists of the norms, criteria, and standards used as measures in the evaluation process (6).

Incorporating the questions of what we are assuring, for whom, how, the domains of structure, process, and outcome, and the variables we will choose to investigate, Wong (5) has come up with a definition which seems applicable within the context of advanced nursing practice. This definition assures the consumer a degree of excellence through an ongoing process of measuring and evaluating the setting and conditions of care, the process of nursing intervention, and/or patient outcomes. It is predicated on using the pre-established criteria and standards. There is no end point to this quality improvement process. Evaluations lead to changes aimed at improving care, and the circle begins again (3).

Instituting a Quality Improvement Program in Advanced Practice

Defining Quality or Excellence

The first step in initiating a program for evaluating care is to define what is meant by excellence for the particular agency, program, managed care system, or practice. It is helpful to review the objectives of the program, if they exist, and to decide if excellence is synonymous with achieving them. Usually, the objectives of an organization, managed care system, or practice are broad enough to achieve consensus among those who will be involved in the quality improvement process. If the agency is a nonprofit, voluntary entity or a community or neighborhood center, there is a good chance that consumers have had input in formulating the objectives. Nurses in independent practice usually predicate their practice on goals related to the benefits they envision their services providing for patients. Some practices are based on community assessment, which yields data on the needs of the target population, and services are directed toward meeting those needs. Finally, managed care systems are setting goals and demanding that their employees meet those goals, many of which have had more to do with billable hours and the bottom line than quality of care for patients. Ideally, the first step in the quality improvement process affords the nurses involved an opportunity to discuss what they perceive as excellence for their practice, which can evolve into a clarification of values. It can help nurses understand where each is coming from and open up communication as differences are revealed. The hazard exists, of course, that being honest about one's values can have the effect of isolating one or more individuals from the group or creating two camps. Chances are, however, that members of the group are aware of differences already. The benefits to be gained through an honest discussion usually outweigh the hazards, particularly when an atmosphere is created that is non-threatening and uncensoring of any opinion.

Quality Improvement—for Whom?

Once an agreement is reached as to the definition of excellence in practice, it is important to discuss for whose benefit the quality improvement program is being launched. If it is to satisfy the requirements for accreditation, licensure, credentialing, or third-party regulations imposed by an official body or agency, then the methods chosen and the domains included should be those most appropriate for that task. Since a health care delivery system purportedly must address the needs of its patients, quality improvement would also necessarily be concerned with assuring a good quality of care for those persons. A quality improvement program might have as its sole purpose accountability to patients, or it might address the agency needs for accountability to accrediting and professional bodies as well. Increasingly, such programs are also demanded by third-party payers. When the highest possible quality of care for patients to assure the best possible outcomes is not the focus or at least a focus of quality improvement, and cost of care assumes greater importance, health care professionals can find themselves caught in the middle.

*Structure, Process, or Outcome**

The next step in establishing a program for quality improvement is to decide on which of the three domains—structure, process, or outcome—to utilize for the process (9). Programs which look at structure might examine components of services such as the setting and the conditions. Some of these components are listed in Table 11.1. The decision as to which domain(s) to include will depend upon the purpose of, and target for, the quality improvement program. Criteria from licensing or accrediting bodies or managed care systems may dictate the domain. If the focus is on quality improvement for patients and total system quality, all three domains may be relevant. Certainly, we as providers are concerned about the structure and process as well as outcomes and patient satisfaction in all three domains.

Criteria, Standards, Norms

Criteria. Once the decision has been made as to the domains to include, the measurement (norms and/or standards) criteria must be set or chosen. A number of examples exist in the literature for criteria, norms, and standards for structure, process, and outcome. It is important to distinguish among these three as variables that might be chosen for examination. According to Bloch (6), a criterion is value free and is the name of a variable either believed or known to be a relevant indicator of the quality of patient care. Criteria may be explicit statements of performance, circumstances, behavior or clinical status. Examples of criteria are included in many publications (7, 8, 9, 10, 11). Table 11.2 gives examples of structure, process, and outcome criteria for advanced practice nurses.

Developing criteria for quality improvement programs is a very difficult task. Information must be obtained, and it is not always possible to find the kind of information from the literature

---

*An alternative model is the Stufflebeam CIPP evaluation model—context, input, process, and product (8).

Table 11.1.   Measurement Domains for Quality Improvement*

STRUCTURE
Philosophy and objectives of agency, program, practice, institution, care
     system
Organizational characteristics
Impact on quality and cost of care
Resources
     fiscal
     equipment
     physical facilities
     personnel
Legal aspects to support mission
Management structure
Licensure, certification, accreditation status, approval, third-party
     regulations
Employees
     qualifications
     goals
     characteristics
     degree of colleagueship
     attitudes and values
     amount and kind of supervision available
Patients
     expectations
     attitudes
Values
     bio0physical and psycho/cultural/social characteristics on entering system

PROCESS
Delivery of nursing care
     type
     behaviors of nurse
     sequence of events
     activities
     degree of skill of providers
Interactions
     among providers
     with patients
     with significant others

(continued)

Table 11.1. (Continued)

inclusion of patient, significant others
Techniques, procedures
Coordination of care
 among different components of the system
 among members of team
 continuity of care across settings
Components of care
 among different components of the system
 among members of team
 continuity of care across settings
Components of the care system
 utilization
 those available

OUTCOME
End results of nursing care
 change in health status
 patient compliance and satisfaction
 change in patient behavior, knowledge of mastery
 mortality
 morbidity
 disability
 social functioning
 activities of daily living

---

* Adapted from Kennedy-Malone (1996). American Nurses Association. (1996). Quality Assurance Workbook, pp. 12-17. Kansas City, MO: American Nurses Association.

---

that is valid and useful for a quality improvement program (12). For example, although one may wish to access information on management strategies and outcome criteria for hypertension control in adults 60 years and older, these data may be difficult to unearth. An extensive review of studies to date may be useful (13).

Establishing reliable criteria includes the following steps: literature search, examining the criteria that already exist; using experience and clinical expertise of those preparing criteria; and a good deal of thinking. Criteria should be based on a nursing model

Table 11.2. Examples of Criteria in the Three Domains

STRUCTURE

National certification is required for each nurse in advanced practice.

The nurse practicing as an advanced practice nurse must be a graduate of an approved certificate or master's program.

The caseload ratio is one nurse for every 350 patients.

Each professional provider is granted a minimum of five days per year for continuing studies.

Peer evaluation within the setting is intra- and interdisciplinary.

All members of the team have an equal voice in decision making for the agency.

Each advanced practice nurse must hold a DEA license and obtain and maintain prescriptive authority

PROCESS

The name and action of the drug will be explained to the patient each time a prescription is written.

Assessment methods will be chosen on the basis of risk factors and patient perception of the problem.

Significant others are included in the caregiving process.

All patient assessments, planning, interventions, and evaluations are recorded using problem oriented format.

A problem list is to be prepared for each patient at the first visit and updated at each subsequent visit.

A minimum of one-half hour will be allowed for each nurse visit and one hour for a first visit assessment.

OUTCOME

The annual rate of hospitalization is reduced in the target population.

Hypertension control as measured by mean blood pressure readings is attained.

Over one year a weight loss pattern will be established for obese patients.

Maintenance of optimal level of wellness for all patients in caseload as demonstrated by ability to perform activities of daily living at or above level of first visit.

for practice (14). Once criteria are developed, a panel of experts canas to their appropriateness for the concepts being measured. Establishing the validity of the criteria is another step in the process. To do this, multiple measures of the same concepts using external criteria can be done (15). Instruments for measuring criteria can be developed. Some examples of this exist in the lit- erature (7, 16, 17), including the Clinical Practice Development Model (18) and the American Association of Critical Care Nurses Certification Corporation Synergy Model (22). A number of measures of quality of care that have been developed for nursing appear in the literature (17, 19, 44).

Standards. Standards may be defined as achievable levels or ranges of performance which correspond with a criterion against which an actual performance may be compared (5). A standard may also be defined as compliance plus or minus a percentage of variance from a norm that is agreed upon as safe or excellent practice (20). A standard may also refer to a level of magnitude on a scale in order to make a statement about the quality of outcomes (20).

The American Nurses Association's standards for nursing prac- tice are examples of standards of excellence for nursing practice that can be adopted or adapted for a practice, agency, or institution. Guides for implementing standards has also been prepared (21). Other organizations such as the Association of Women's Health, Obstetric, and Neonatal Nurses, National Association of Pediatric Nurse Practitioners Associates (NAPNAP), the American College of Nurse Midwives, and the American Association of Nurse Anesthe- tists have also developed standards and some of these appear in Appendix A.

Norms. A norm is a range or level of performance. It is generally the current "one" unless otherwise stated, and is generated from a descriptive investigation of a particular population, region, community, or group (6). Another definition of a norm describes it as a prevailing pattern or percentage of compliance (20). Norms may be statistical measures that are generated from a large data pool (21).

Mechanisms

Finally, methods must be chosen for the process of quality improvement. Audits, peer reviews, chart reviews, postcare patient interviews or questionnaires, and staff conferences are some of the mechanisms that are employed (20). Methods for concurrent evaluation include open chart audits, patient interviews and observations, interviewing and/or observing staff, and conferences of caregivers (7, 20, 21). Each of these methods might be appropriate for the advanced practice nurse. Examples of ways to implement each of these mechanisms can be found in Table 11.3.

Audit. "Audit" is an umbrella term to mean the process of judging, retrospectively, the quality of nursing care with reference to professional standards. The audit has come to be synonymous with a retrospective chart review, the method generally used to obtain information on the "achievement, trends, and problems" for those under care (23, p. 31). The audit gathers data on the patient and setting, and a random sample of patient records is chosen for review. A quality score is given along with remarks by the reviewer focusing on policy, procedures, and practices (23, p. 35).

Outcome criteria can be used in the audit process (21). In ambulatory care with a long-term caseload, a retrospective audit might be done on a random sample of patients at the end of one year. Outcome criteria in relation to factors such as hypertension control, fertility control, weight loss or gain, and maintenance or restoration of the ability to perform activities of daily living might be evaluated as part of the audit. Audits can also use the standards of care prepared by professional organizations as criteria. Phaneuf (23) also suggests using Lesnik and Anderson's 7 functions of nursing: application and execution of physician's legal orders as appropriate; observations of signs, symptoms and reactions; supervision of patient; supervision of those who participate in care (except physicians) or acting as case manager for a multidisciplinary team; reporting and recording; application and execution of nursing procedures and techniques; and promotion of physical and emotional health through direction and teaching (24). Some of these are applic-

---

Table 11.3   Mechanisms for Quality Improvement in Nursing Care Settings

Mechanisms	*Examples*
Chart audit and review	Retrospective: pull charts randomly from file of patients not seen in last 6 months and identify strengths and deficits of care based on documentation in records.
	Open Chart: review of chart against predetermined criteria and feedback to caregiver.
	Group Audit: intra- or interdisciplinary, of randomly selected charts representing patients cared for by one or more team members; review again predetermined criteria and critique of care.
	Independent Solo Practice: - Review of records with peer or peers consulting on a regular basis.
Patient interview and inspection	Specific interview and assessment as part of care process. Elicit subjective and objective data on patient perception of structure and process as well as outcome.
Postcare questionnaires	Instruments designed to elicit perceptions of structures, process, and/or outcome from patients' perceptions. May be filled out after a visit with a caregiver or at the end of a given time a patient is in a particular practice or agency.
Utilization of instruments for measuring specific variables	Patient assessment guides. Problem lists with outcome criteria and scoring system for these.
Staff interview or observation	Peer or interdisciplinary observation of the interview interactional process between provider and patient; feedback after visit is over.

(continued)____

Table 11.3   (continued)

Mechanisms	*Examples*
Group conferencing - concurrent domains.	Inter- or intradisciplinary case review of selected patients; may also involve patient, family, significant others. Focus may be on any or all of the three
Postcare conferencing	Review of selected patient cases no longer in caseload; involve all members of team who participated in care.
Postcare patient interviews	Interview patient or group of patients after discharge from care system. In ambulatory setting, could be after a crisis and crisis resolution.

able to the advanced practice nurse's clinical activities; others are not, or would need modification. An example of an audit tool for nursing appears in Table 11.4.

In one example of audit for an ambulatory unit, charts for 25 patients who had visited an obstetric clinic over the past 12 months were randomly selected. Data were retrieved and all staff participated in the review. The audit was carried out following methods developed by the Medical Quality Assurance Committee of the Joint Commission for the Accreditation of Health Care Organizations (JCAHO)—the Performance Evaluation Procedure for Auditing and Improving Patient Care (PEP) (25).

Another example of the use of audit comes from a public health nursing agency. This agency used as criteria seven nursing functions and made judgments on a five-point scale from "Excellent" to "Unsafe" for each case audited through record review. The cases were clustered as to primary medical diagnoses (26). The results were then communicated by the nursing audit committee through supervisors to the staff nurses. The audit was considered to be one tool to appraise the quality of services (26).

Thus, the audit can be one mechanism used for a quality im-

Table 11.4. **Example of Audit Tool for Nursing Setting***

Patient's name: _____

_____Patient's sex: _____ Age: _____ Date of last Visit:_____

_____Number of visits in past 12 months: _____

_____Nursing diagnosis: _____

_____

_____Hazardous events (biophysical and psychosocial)

situational: _____

_____ developmental: _____

_____Hospitalizations in past 12 months: _____

_____Nursing visits signed and identified: _____

_____Problem list completed and updated to last visit: _____**Audit Criteria:**

*Adapted from Phaneuf, 1976, Appendix 3(26); Dorsey and Hussa, 1979, (29) pp. 41-43.

---

provement program. It has both advantages and limitations. A retrospective record audit assesses the quality of the record rather than of the care given. Setting criteria and standards is a difficult task. Rating scales are difficult to construct and by their very nature impose value judgments. Words which may be chosen, such as "good," "excellent," and "poor," have value-laden connotations.

Quality of nursing care is one facet of an interactional process involving patient, perhaps family and/or significant others, and at times the community and other health care providers. Validity is dependent upon professional judgments. Reliability of judgments can be tested by experts in practice. Some of the knotty problems of using audit include who should do it and to what end. Although intended to be educational and constructive, audit may end up being used for purposes that tend to be punitive and destructive. Once the results of audit are ready, they must be used to improve care or the purpose of the process is lost. If change is short-lived, has the audit lost its purpose? How effective are attempts to effect change in professional behavior? The costs of the audit also must be considered. Are the ends worth the means? Is it a cost effective process? Does it achieve its purpose? (27).

The value of the audit to nurses can be multidimensional. It can bring about change in awareness, in perceptions of care, in knowledge, and in abilities. It can also serve as a consciousness-raising experience. If nurses have input into the process of developing criteria, factual knowledge can accrue. Audits also help to emphasize the role of nursing in patient care and the independent nursing diagnoses and management strategies that are possible. The results of patient teaching become apparent through the evaluation process.

Since a search of the literature is necessary for developing criteria, staff are exposed to and can have an opportunity to discuss current research and practices. The audit process can also generate research as a spin-off. Queries that arise as to definitions of nursing practice or the validity of management strategies can generate research questions.

Feedback affords nurses the opportunity to consider goals for patient care and to evaluate reasons for failure to document care. An audit also reinforces the need for accountability through documentation. What has the potential of being a threatening process can be turned into a positive learning opportunity (28).

Peer Review. Peer review is the process by which a group of nursing colleagues evaluates the effectiveness of the work of its peers. Prior to implementing the process, criteria for the evaluation are developed. Criteria are then applied to an actual patient care situation (29). (See Appendix C.)

Peer review has been suggested as an integral part of developing the roles of advanced nurses (29). Peer review may also be interdisciplinary, as among members of a health care team such as might exist in a community health center or in outpatient clinics. For the nurse working in solo practice, peer review can be arranged through consultation with advanced practitioners working in similar settings. Peer review can be ongoing or periodic. It can be based on the standards of care and the scope of practice developed through professional organizations or upon criteria established for a particular practice or care system agency (29). Peer review can be conducted in a number of ways. One of these is chart audit and review. Another is through direct observation of a patient care episode followed by an evalu-ation. The nurse being reviewed may present a patient case or selected patients from her/his caseload for review.

Peer review for advanced practice nurses can include evaluation of nurse-developed protocols, knowledge and management strategies, incorporation of education, philosophy of practice, and patient feedback. Forms can be developed for the review process and used for evaluating and sharing sessions and as a guide for improving care (29). An example of a peer review form can be found in Table 11.5. Another example is described and evaluated in the work of Goodwin, Jacox, Prescott and colleagues (30, 31, 32).

As with any evaluation process, there are both advantages and some pitfalls. There are satisfactions to be gained from documenting the health care nurses are providing. Nurses also can gain an awareness of the importance of developing instruments to measure components of health care. Quality of care can be improved. For the nurse working in an isolated area or as the only advanced practice nurse in a care setting, peer review provides a mechanism for sharing knowledge and experience (33). Peer review is one method for implementing standards of practice and for controlling practice within the profession (34). Peer review encourages examination of self and one's own practice. It can serve to encourage self-study and continuing education. Levels of competence are identified (29).

Peer review has some pitfalls as well. It can be anxiety-producing and threatening. There is a temptation to engage in "in-group self-protection" at the expense of the public (34). There is also a danger that interests in economic welfare of the system, especially if it operates for profit, will usurp interests in quality and cost of care

Table 11.5   Peer Review Worksheet

Nurse:_____ Reviewer: _____
Setting:_____ Date of review: _____
A. Protocols (developed by nurse*)
    Literature
    Type
    Appropriateness of management strategies
    Evaluation tool
B. Colleague interaction
    Use of referrals
    Collaboration with other nurses—peer consultation
    Collaboration and coordination with other providers
    Chart review and results
C. Nurse knowledge and preparation
    Continuing education: when, what?
    Journals read regularly
    Examples of knowledge of current research and application in
       practice
    Engaged in research at present? If so, what?
    Record keeping
       Complete?
       POMR or other record keeping system
       Reflective of appropriate management strategies
       Patient education - documentation
D. Observations
    Interactions: appropriate, quality
    Nursing process
    Patient assessment, planning, intervention, evaluation
    Charting reflective of process
    Plans for follow-up
    Measure of patient satisfaction with care
E. Nurse's philosophy: ability to articulate; familiarity with scope of
    practice, standards of care; model for practice; state legal and
    regulatory statutes for advance practice
Comments of nurse:
Comments of reviewer:
Plans based on assessment:

*And approved by physician colleague if required by nurse practice act.

(34). Peer review cannot be forced on any nurse. It will not be effective if the nurse does not see it as her/his responsibility and right (35). Time and distance can be inhibiting factors, especially in rural areas (33). *Interviews and Questionnaires.* These can be used to elicit input as to patients' perceptions of care (43). Interviewing is more flexible and has a higher response rate than questionnaires, although it is a more expensive method. Also, responses may reflect the patient's attempts to please the interviewer (36).

Questionnaires can assure confidentiality and are less costly and time-consuming than interviews. They are especially useful when geographic distribution is great. They can be handed out at the end of a visit or mailed to a sample of patients. However, the response rate is usually low, items may be skipped, and there is usually no opportunity to elicit further information. The respondents' level of understanding and language must be taken into account (36). The use of a computer should be considered when constructing the instrument. An example of an evaluation questionnaire appears in Table 11.6.

Patient feedback is important, if not critical, to the health care delivery process. Input reflects the opinions of patients and can thus help nurses improve public relations, foster morale among providers, and dispel tensions between patients and care givers (37). Feedback to the patient following the evaluation will help to facilitate communication and encourage openness.

Some agencies also hold an open group meeting periodically for the purposes of review and evaluation. Patients can then meet with members of the caregiving team (37). This could be done both for individual patients and for a group.

Summary

Quality improvement is an important component of the caregiving process. Accountability to consumers is increasing in importance as demands are voiced and is already, in many cases, tied to third-party reimbursement for services. Several tasks remain in the on-going process of developing models for improvement programs for

----

Table 11.6 Patient Questionnaire

In order to improve our services, we would appreciate your taking a few minutes to answer the following questions.

1. When you came for your appointment, were you generally well-received and treated courteously by the staff?
   Yes _____ No _____

2. Once at your appointment, how long did you wait to be seen?
   Less than 15 minutes _____ 15-30 minutes _____
   30-60 minutes _____ Over an hour _____

3. How would you rate the competence of the nurse practitioner who saw you in meeting your needs?
   Outstanding _____ Above average _____ Average _____
   Below average _____ Way below average _____

4. How would you rate the explanation of examination procedures and care you received?
   Outstanding _____ Above average _____ Average _____
   Below average _____ Way below average _____

5. How would you rate the concern of the nurse practitioner with your feelings as a person?
   Outstanding _____ Above average _____ Average _____
   Below average _____ Way below average _____

6. Do you think such concern is appropriate as part of care?
   Always _____ Almost always _____ Sometimes _____
   Rarely _____ Never _____

7. Did your problem require consultation with a physician or other health care provider?   Yes _____ No _____

8. If not, did you wish to see a physician or other health care provider?
   Yes _____ No _____

(continued)

Table 11.6 (continued)

9. Did other caregivers participate in your care (receptionist, lab technician, X-ray technician, nurse, nursing assistant)?
   Yes ____ No ____
   If so, did all of these persons identify themselves to you and/or wear name badges?   Yes ____ No ____

10. Prior to this visit, how many times have you had a health exam as an adult?
    Never ____ Once ____ More than once ____

11. If you answered "Once" or "More than once" to Question 9, where was the exam (exams) performed?
    Physician's office or clinic ____
    This setting ____ Other care setting (such as a hospital emergency department, HMO) ____

12. If you have been to other health care services settings, how would you compare care in this setting with those other clinics?
    Much better ____ Better ____ Equal to ____
    Worse ____ Much worse ____

13. In the future, if you have similar health care needs, would you prefer to see:
    An advanced practice nurse ____ A physician ____
    Doesn't matter ____

14. Please add any suggestions or comments concerning health care.

Thank you! Your cooperation will help us to serve you better.

advanced practice nursing. We need to continue to develop outcome criteria for patients. Nursing also needs to develop nursing care and management-specific outcome criteria. Bloch (38) has suggested establishing a national clearinghouse on nursing evaluation to foster coordination and the sharing of ideas and to avoid duplication of work. This center could also establish a list of experts and consultants.

In the new millennium, it is evident that the role of regulation in quality improvement will become paramount (39). It would behoove the nursing profession to take the lead in defining quality nursing care and in publicly embracing the role of CQI in nursing practice (40). Several quality improvement programs and efforts to incorporate the principles of CQI into nursing care delivery have been underway since the 1980s (41, 42, 43, 44). We have come a long way from assigning blame to individuals for mistakes to where we now use a process analysis to improve the system of care delivery (45, 46). Nevertheless, the CQI movement has not made a sizable impact on the US health care system (40). Until there is wide-spread recognition of the need for drastic change, universal commitment to CQI principles will not be achieved (41).

Advanced practitioners must take the lead in redefining the system that rewards nurses for professional excellence in quality improvement in patient care. Advanced practice nurses must incorporate QI principles and tools in daily practice. Our time has come: CQI is a breakthrough where advanced practice nurses can demonstrate a major positive impact on quality and cost-effective health care delivery for the future (49).

REFERENCES

1.   Bailit, H., Lewis, J., Hochheiser, L., & Bush, N. (1975). Assessing the quality of care. *Nursing Outlook 23:153-159.*
1a   Malone, B.L. (1986). Evaluation of the clinical nurse specialist. *American Journal of Nursing 86:1375-1377.*
1b   Ingersoll, G.L. (1988). Evaluating the impact of a clinical nurse specialist. *Clinical Nurse Specialist 2(3):150-155.*
2.   Zimmer, M.J. (1974). Quality assurance for outcomes of patient care. *Nursing Clinics of North America 9:305-315.*
3.   Kirk, R. (1992). The big picture: Total quality management and continuous quality improvements. *Journal of Nursing Administration 22:24-31.*
4.   Juran, J.M. (1989). *Juran on Leadership for Quality: An Executive Handbook.* New York: The Free Press, p. 28.
5.   Wong, S.T. (1998). Outcomes of nursing care: How do we know? *Clinical*

Nurse Specialist 12(4):147-151.

6. Bloch, D. (1977). Criteria, standards, norms - crucial terms in quality assurance. *Journal of Nursing Administration 1:22, 26.*

7. AWHONN (1998). *Achieving Consistent Quality Care: Using Evidence to Guide Practice.* Washington, DC: AWHONN

8. Kennedy-Malone, L.M. (1996). Evaluation strategies for CNSs: Application of an evaluation model. *Clinical Nurse Specialist 10(4):195-198.*

9. McAlpine, L.A. (1997). Process and outcome measures for the multidisciplinary collaborative projects of a critical care CNS. *Clinical Nurse Specialist 11(3):134-138.*

10. Barnason, S., Merboth, M., Pozehl, B. & Tietjen, M.J. (1998). Utilizing an outcomes approach to improve pain management by nurses: A pilot study. *Clinical Nurse Specialist 12(1):28-36.*

11. Olsson, U., Bergbon-Engberg, I. & Ahs, M. (1998). Evaluating nurses' knowledge and patients' energy after intervention. *Clinical Nurse Specialist 12(6):217-225.*

12. Williamson, J.W. (1980). Information management in quality assurance. *Nursing Research 29:78-81.*

13. Lang, N.M. & Marek, K.D. (1992). Outcomes that reflect clinical practice. *Proceedings of a Conference Sponsored by the National Center for Nursing Research.* Patient outcomes research: Examining the effectiveness of nursing practice. Report No. 93-3411.

14. Runtz, S.F. & Urtel, J.G. (1983). Evaluating your practice via a nursing model. *Nurse Practitioner 8:30, 32, 37-40.*4

15. Horn, B.J. (1980). Establishing valid and reliable criteria: A researcher's perspective. *Nursing Research 29:88-90.*

16. Dienemann, J. (Ed.) (1993). *Continuous Quality Improvement in Nursing.* Washington, DC: American Nurses Publishing.

17. Rantz, M.J. (1990): *Nursing Quality Measurement: A Review of Nursing Studies.* Washington, DC: American Nurses Publishing.

18. Haag-Heitman, B. & Kramer, A. (1998). Creating a clinical practice development model. *American Journal of Nursing 98(8):39-43.*

19. American Nurses Association. (1995). *Nursing Care Report Card for Acute Care.* Washington, DC: American Nurses Publishing.

20. American Nurses Association. (1996). *Nursing Quality Indicators: Definitions and Implications.* Washington, DC: American Nurses Publishing.

21. American Nurses Association. (1996). *Nursing Quality Indicators: Guide for Implementation.* Washington, DC: American Nurses Publishing.

22. Curley, M.A.Q. (1998). Patient-nurse synergy: Optimizing patients' outcomes. *American Journal of Critical Care 7(1):64-72.*

23. Phaneuf, M.C. (1976). *The Nursing Audit* (2nd ed.). New York: Appleton-Century-Crofts. p. 3.

24. Lesnik, M.J. & Anderson, B.E. (1955). *Nursing Practice and the Law.* Philadelphia: J.B. Lippincott. pp. 259-260.

25. Dorsey, B. & Hussa, R.K. (1979). Evaluating ambulatory care: Three approaches. *Journal of Nursing Administration 74:24-35.*

26. Phaneuf, M.C. (1969). Quality of care: Problems of measurement. Am-

erican Journal of Public Health 59:1829-1831.

27.   Donabedian, A. (1969). Some issues in evaluating the quality of nursing care. *American Journal of Public Health 59:1833-1836.*

28.   Moore, K.R. (1979). What nurses learn from nursing audit. *Nursing Outlook 27:254-258.*

29.   Komelasky, A.L., Bridgers, C., Golas, G., Pence, D. & Woodard, I. (1997). Developing a peer review system: One HMO's experience. *Advance for Nurse Practitioners 2(1):73-77.*

30.   Goodwin, L., Prescott, P., Jacox, A., & Collar, M. (1981). The nurse practitioner rating scale II. *Nursing Research 30:270-276.*

31.   Prescott, P.A., Jacox, A., Collar, M. & Goodwin, L. (1981). The nurse practitioner rating form I. *Nursing Research 30:223-228.*

32.   Jacox, A., Prescott, P., Collar, M. & Goodwin, L. (1981). *A Primary Care Process Measure. The Nurse Practitioner Rating Form.* Wakefield, MA: Nursing Resources.

33.   Hiserote, J.L., Bultemeier, K., Kimberly, S.L., Nicoll, J.C. & Wheeler, K. (1980). Peer review among rural clinics. *The Nurse Practitioner 5:30-32.*

34.   Ramphal, M. (1974). Peer review. *American Journal of Nursing 74:63-67.*

35.   Hauser, M.A. (1975). Initiation into peer review. *American Journal of Nursing 75:2204-2207.*

36.   Marriner, A. (1979). The research process in quality assurance. *American Journal of Nursing 79:2158-2161.*

37.   Froebe, D.J. & Bain, R.J. (1976). *Quality Assurance Programs and Controls in Nursing.* St. Louis: C.V. Mosby. pp. 81-82.

38.   Bloch, D. (1975). Evaluation of nursing care in terms of process and outcome: Issues in research and quality assurance. *Nursing Research 4:256-263.*

39.   Brennan, T.A. (1998). The role of regulation in quality improvement. *Millbank Quarterly 76(4):709-731.*

40.   Strange, R. (1998). Homing in on quality. *Elder Care 10(4):17-20.*

41.   Barton, A. & Danek, G. (1998). Improving patient outcomes through CQI: Vascular access planning. *Journal of Nursing Care Quality 13(2):77-85.*

42.   Brisco, C.G. & Arthur, G. (1998). CQI teamwork: Reevaluate, restructure, renew. *Nursing Management 29(10):73-80.*

49.   Koch, M.W. (1991). Continuous quality improvement implications for nursing administration. The facilitator. Council on Nursing Administration, ANA: Kansas City, MO: 17:4-6.

43.   Hetherington, L.R. (1998). Evaluating quality management systems. *Journal of Nursing Care Quality 13(2):56-66.*

44.   Massarweh, L.J. (1998). TQM in critical care. *Nursing Management 29(6):480-481.*

45.   Lepley, C.J. (1999). Problem-solving tools for analyzing system problems. The affinity map and the relationship diagram. *Journal of Nursing Administration 28(12):44-50.*

46.   Blumenthal, D. & Kilo, M. (1998). A report card on continuous quality improvement. *Millbank Quarterly 76(4):635-648.*

47. Darling, H. (1998). Continuous Quality Improvement: Does it matter? *Millbank Quarterly 76(4):755-757.*

BIBLIOGRAPHY

Aguayo, R. (1990). Dr. Deming. *The American Who Taught the Japanese about Quality.* New York: Carol Publishing Group.

American Nurses Association. (1995). *Quality: The State of the Art of Nursing Quality Management.* Washington DC: American Nurses Publishing.

Anderson-Loftin, W., Wood, D. & Whitfield, L. (1995). A case study of nursing care management in a rural hospital. *Nursing Administration Quarterly 19(3):33-40.*

Arikan, V.L. (1991). Total quality management: Applications to nursing service. *Journal of Nursing Administration 21:46-50.*

Arnold, M.C. (1994). A quality improvement program for a clinical nurse specialist department. *Journal of Nursing Care Quality 8(44):42-47.*

Avis, M., Bond, M. & Arthur, A. (1997). Questioning patient satisfaction: An empirical investigation in two outpatient clinics. *Social Science & Medicine 44:85-92.*

Barnason, S., Merboth, M., Pozehl, B. & Tietjen, M.J. (1998). Utilizing an outcomes approach to improve pain management by nurses: A pilot study. *Clinical Nurse Specialist 12:28-36.*

Casalou, R. (1991). Total quality management in health care. *Hospitals & Health Services Administration 36:134-146.*

Courtney, R. & Rice, C. (1997). Investigation of nurse practitioner-patient interactions: Using the nurse practitioner rating form. *Nurse Practitioner 22:46-65.*

Deming, W.E. (1986). *Out of the Crisis.* Cambridge, MA: Institute of Technology Center for Advanced Engineering Study.

Dempsey, C. (1995). Nursing home acquired pneumonia: Outcomes from a clinical process improvement program. *Pharmacotherapy 15:335-385.*

Evans, M.L., Martin, M.L. & Winslow, E.H. (1998). Nursing care and patient satisfaction. *American Journal of Nursing 98(12):57-59.*

Gillem, T.R. (1988).Deming's 14 points and hospital quality: Responding to the consumer's demand for the best value in health care. *Nursing Quality Assurance 2:70-80.*

Gitlow, H E. & Gitlow, S. (1987). *The Deming Guide to Quality and Competitive Position.* Englewood, NJ: Prentice-Hall.

Houston, S. & Fletcher, R. (1997). Outcomes management in women's health. *Journal of Obstetric, Gynecologic, and Neonatal Nursing 26:342-350.*

Houston, S. & Luquire, R. (1991). Measuring success: CNS performance appraisal. *Clinical Nurse Specialist 5(4):204-209.*

Howard, J. & Wolff, P. (1992). Evaluation of clinical nurse specialist practice. *Clinical Nurse Specialist 6(1):28-35.*

Jones, K.R., Jenning, B.M., Moritz, P. & Moss, M.T. (1997). Policy issues associated with analyzing outcomes of care. *Image 29:261-267.*

Kearnes, D.R. (1992). A productivity tool to evaluate NP practice: Monitoring clinical time spent in reimbursable patient-related activities. *The Nurse Practitioner 17(4):50; 52; 55.*

Kirk, R. & Hoesing, H. (1991). *Common Sense Quality Management: The Nurse's Guide.* West Dundee, IL: S/N Publications.

Kleinpell, R.M. & Piano, M.R. (Eds.) (1998). *Practice Issues for the Acute Care Nurse Practitioner.* New York: Springer.

Kovner, C. & Gergen, P.J. (1998). Nursing staff levels and adverse events following surgery in U.S. hospitals. *Image 30(4):315-321.*

Lanza, M.L. (1997). Feminist leadership through total quality management. *Health Care for Women International 8:95-106.*

Leming, T. (1991). Quality customer service: Nursing's new challenge. *Nursing Administration Quarterly 15:6-12.*

Martin, J.P. (1989). From implication to reality through a unit-based quality assurance program. *Clinical Nurse Specialist 3(4):192-196.*

Mitchell, P.H., Ferketich, S., Jennings, B.M. & American Academy of Nursing Expert Panel on Quality Health Care. (1998). *Quality health outcomes model. Image 30:43-46.*

Morin, G. (1995). A personal performance checklist. *Nursing Management 26(2):32C, 32G.*

Mullin, M.H., Opperwall, B.C. & White, S.L. (1995). CNS development of health maintenance programs: Quality improvement and cost reduction. *Clinical Nurse Specialist 9:45-49.*

Naylor, M.D., Munro, B.H. & Brooten, D.A. (1991). Measuring the effectiveness of nursing practice. *Clinical Nurse Specialist 5(4):210-215.*

Noll, M.L. & Girard, N. (1993). Preparing the CNS for participation in quality assurance activities. *Clinical Nurse Specialist 7:81-84.*

Nugent, K.E. & Lambert, V.A. (1997). Evaluating the performance of the APN. *Nurse Practitioner 22:190-198.*

Peglow, D., Klatt-Ellis, T., Stelton, S., et al. (1992). Evaluation of clinical nurse specialist practice. *Clinical Nurse Specialist 6(1):28-35.*4

Shindul-Rothschild, J., Long-Middleton, E. & Berry, D. (1997). 10 keys to quality care. *American Journal of Nursing 97(11):35-43.*

Stone, P.W. & Walker, P.H. (1997). Clinical and cost outcomes of a free-standing birth center:A comparison study. *Clinical Excellence for Nurse Practitioners 1(7):456-465.*

Waltz, C.F. & Sylvia, B.M. (1991). Accountability and outcome measurement: Where do we go from here? *Clinical Nurse Specialist 5(4):202-203.*

Wong, S.T., Bernick, L.A., Portillo, C., et al. (1999). Implementing a nurse information system in a nurse-managed primary care practice: A process in progress. *Clinical Excellence for Nurse Practitioners: The International Journal of NPACE 3(2):123-127.*

Zonsius, M. & Murphy, M. (1995). Use of total quality management sparks staff nurse participation in continuous quality improvement. *Nursing Clinics of North America 30(1):1-2.*

ONLINE RESOURCES

Healthcare quality improvement resources, information relating to JCAHO accreditation surveys: **www.hqir.com**

Healthy People 2010: **web.health.gov/healthypeople**

Multiple government and business resources for CQI, recent article, references, and extensive bibliography: **www.iqd.com**

University of Texas at Houston Health Science web page offering CQI initiatives, budget suggestions, tools, staff development:
www.uth.tmc.edu

AHCPR website for quality assessment: **http://www.ahcpr.gov**

12

Community Assessment

Introduction

From the inception of advanced practice roles for nurses with the first nurse anesthetists in 1877, followed shortly thereafter with public health nurses and then nurse-midwives, clinical nurse specialists, and nurse practitioners, these nurses have been pioneers and mavericks. When surgeons began to use anesthesia, the mortality rate was unacceptably high. Because of this and because the pay for administering anesthesia was low, physicians were not interested in this specialty, but nurses were and some became nurse anesthetists (1). Public health nurses brought care to tenement dwellers in cities and, beginning with the establishment of school nursing in New York City in 1902, to school children (2, 4). Nurse-midwives changed the morbidity and mortality rates for infants and mothers in Kentucky and for tenement women and babies in cities, including New York and Chicago (5, 6). Nurse practitioners improved the availability of health care to city and rural residents through community and rural health centers (3, 9, 10). Clinical nurse specialists have made psychiatric mental health care available to more persons through community mental health clinics, and now through manage care systems and in specialty and general hospitals, but long before this role was conceptualized, nurses received special preparation to care for the mentally ill in training schools located in specialty hospitals such as Butler Hospital in Providence, Rhode Island, and Worcester State Hospital in Worcester, Massachusetts (23, 24). What these nurses with advanced practice skills have in common is their ability to identify needs in a community and create ways to meet them.

The concept of nursing's involvement in community assessment is not unique to the roles of advanced practice nurses today. Early in this century, Lillian Wald observed the needs of the poor in New York City and took steps to meet those needs through expanding the role of public health nurses and establishing the Henry Street Settlement (4). She also saw a need for a stronger commitment to the health and welfare of the children of this country and, in so doing, was instrumental in founding the Children's Bureau in 1912 (5). In 1925, Mary Breckinridge, recognizing the unmet needs of children and their families in the Kentucky mountains, founded the Frontier Nursing Service (6). As a social worker, Jane Addams saw the need for nursing care for families in the neighborhood surrounding Hull House in the Chicago of the late nineteenth and early twentieth centuries. When the Visiting Nurse Association of Chicago was founded, Hull House was chosen as a site for one of its district substations (7).

Taylor, in a call to advanced practice nurses to envision and implement our preferred future, writes that, "Inherent in nursing activism is the formation of community partnerships and empowerment. . ."(3). Community assessment is a formal means to identify inadequately served, underserved, or ignored communities that nurses might empower through a dialogue about the community's needs.

Conducting a Community Assessment

Our heritage as providers of health care to outcast and underserved groups is as old as nursing and marks us as providers who are sensitive and responsive to the changing needs of our patients. Community assessment is a consequence of the evolving roles of nurses as health care professionals responsible for the needs of individuals, families, and groups within a community and sometimes the whole community.

The focus of practice for an advanced practice nurse should extend beyond the confines of her/his own caseload or immediate setting. Using strategies for community assessment, the nurse engaged in an advanced practice role can identify groups ignored or alienated by traditional means of health care delivery. "Primary health care nurses seek out individuals and groups in need, work with others to uncover poor health conditions, and work with the community at large to bring about needed change" (8).

There are three instances where conducting a community assessment constitutes part of the role of the advanced practice nurse: 1) as part of an already existing agency or institution to ascertain that the providers are meeting the needs of those they serve; 2) prior to creating a new practice or service; and 3) as an attempt to expand or change services or reach out to a changing community.

Who are the groups toward whom nurses might turn their attention in designing a community assessment? Milio (9) identifies these as the poor, those who live in less than desirable locations, ethnic and racial minorities, women, and the aged. These people "lack access to social resources compared to those in the more dominant race, sex, age, income, or geographical groupings." To these we can add the homeless, persons with mental illness, victims of domestic violence, school and day care children and their families, and persons with AIDS. Frontier areas have been designated as areas having less than six persons per square mile when those persons have a lower health status than other rural citizens. These areas offer a special challenge and opportunity to advanced practitioners (10, 30). Developing the role of the clinical nurse specialist with Native Americans is another example of an underserved group on whom advanced practitioners might focus (11). Establishing school-based health centers or centers for advanced practice within established health care institutions are other possibilities (25, 26, 27).

Target groups for health and wellness care within the scope of nursing management might include workers in their places of employment, senior citizens, and members of unions (12, 28). Assessments with potential patient groups or communities might take place in union halls, retirement housing complexes, senior citizen centers, day care centers, the work place, social organizations, schools, and among consumers, self-help groups, and residents of rural areas.

When making an assessment, all available data should be considered in order to get as complete and accurate a picture as possible. To conduct an assessment with a community, a number of methods may be employed. These include observation, interviews, focus groups, community meetings, surveys, use of demographic data, and visits to official agencies such as health departments (local, county, or state), local school districts, police departments, the local health department, and community agencies including the visiting nurse service, senior citizen centers and housing, schools, churches and synagogues, and the local or regional Red Cross chapter. Demographic data are available from these and from local and state disease registries, newspaper files, and census sources (13, 29).

Prior to collecting data, formulate a plan for the assessment, including data management. Computer resources make data collecting, organizing, and managing easier (14). Prepare a purpose and objectives. It is important to be clear about what you wish to find out before approaching individuals or agencies for assistance. Are you planning for a nurse-managed practice and assessing for potential patients? Are you part of a group of advanced practice nurses within or outside a health care agency or institution seeking new opportunities for practice? Is your agency seeking rural health clinic status? Is your agency or community applying for extramural funding? Do you or your agency wish to ascertain the needs of the surrounding community or its desire for new services, or is the assessment aimed at reaffirming your or your agency's role in the community? The cost of doing an assessment must be considered. Who will pay for it? Is a health care agency prepared to cover costs? Can private or public sources be tapped?

List all the possible sources of data required and plan strategies for data collection. Town, county, and state census data can be helpful. Data maintained by schools, courts, police departments, hospitals, health maintenance organizations, other managed care organizations, community health centers, voluntary health-related agencies, community organizations, commercial health-related groups such as Weight Watchers, Diet Workshop, social and fraternal groups, churches, synagogues, as well as those agencies and institutions responsible for direct delivery of health care should not be overlooked if they can contribute information for the assessment (15, 22). "Key informants" are important sources. These may include local housing inspectors, school nurses, public health and parish nurses, welfare and social workers, consumers, members of the local health board, town officials, state senators and representatives, and directors of such groups as Alcoholics Anonymous (15). An up-to-date map is useful if the assessment covers a geographic area of consequence. Use contacts to gain access to those whom you hope to serve if you need their input. For example, a community health center may wish to survey the health needs of all adults over 60 years of age living in a particular town, county, or demarcated area within a city. Using census data, it is possible to estimate the number of such persons and where they reside. To have access to them, unless it is possible to make door-to-door visits, you next need to find out if and where they congregate. Is there a senior citizen's center in the area? Or a parish church with a large proportion of elders? Since visiting nurse or public health nursing services exist in most areas, meet with these providers, explain your purpose, and elicit help.

If your target population consists of working persons, locate all the work places within the geographic area you have defined, then identify a contact person in each place of work. If a Chamber of Commerce exists for the area, you might begin there. Labor unions can also assist you in identifying groups of workers and in providing data on health benefits or services presently in place.

The assessment may focus on the population served by a particular agency, a unit within that agency, a neighborhood, an institution within the community, or the community as a whole. In some cases, an assessment may constitute a research project seeking data to support or reject hypotheses.

If an agency is seeking rural health clinic status in order to qualify for provider reimbursement under the Rural Health Clinics

Act, a community assessment is one step in the approval process (16).

In his book, *Community Health Assessment,* Hanchett (17) has developed a tool kit for community health assessment based on general systems theory, which represents one approach. This book identifies the important components, or subsystems, of the system a community represents, tells how to assess those subsystems which are critical to the study, and offers guidelines for identifying relationships and their attributes. An instrument or instruments for assessing the needs of a community could be developed from the material presented.

In doing a needs assessment, Cordes (15) points out that the difference between need and demand should be considered. He also urges that expected outcomes from meeting health care needs be identified as well as measurable indicators of health care needs. He defines needs as services that should be available regardless of economics and demand as an economic concept. The social costs of particular health risks should also be considered in the assessment process and measured so that these data can be considered in setting priorities on health care planning (15).

After the data collection has been completed, data must be organized, tabulated, analyzed, and a report written or prepared in order to share and preserve the information. The report should include purpose and objectives for the community assessment, how and what data were collected, the findings, and the recommendations. From the report it is possible to generate an action plan with measurable outcome criteria.

Using a Nursing Model for a Community Assessment

Using a nursing model to structure a community assessment from a nursing perspective has several advantages. First, it provides a framework not only for the assessment process, but also for the development of a program of intervention based on findings from the assessment. Second, it forms the basis for nursing practice. Third, it is a framework from which to generate research questions as a component of delivery of care. Records for patients and protocols for the nursing community can evolve from the model. Evaluation tools to monitor the quality of care and patient satisfaction can also be generated through the model. Some interesting debate has resulted from the question of whether or not to base a community assessment on a nursing model (29).

Ford (18) urges that if we want roles as providers of primary care, we must develop components of health care delivery which are superior to those offered by other health care providers. She emphasizes the need to use "an educative-behavioral model of practice rather than a medical one, if we are practicing nursing." Lytle (19) points out that nurses have only recently begun to produced descriptions of services they can offer to patients. The implication is that we need to do far more documentation to provide data to support our role as health care providers and as a basis for accountability. Wellness, assessment and interventions, caring, comforting, teaching, counseling, and coordinating are functions Mauksch (20) identifies as appropriate for nurses, and should be part of a nursing model for practice, but are not a major part of the medical model which focuses on illness, diagnosis, treatment, and curing. While each of these three leaders was speaking or writing almost a quarter of a century ago, their views are timely, given the current chaos in health care. Using a model for nursing practice as a framework for a community assessment might, therefore, seem appropriate. The examples that follow demonstrate the use of the model. It should be noted that this model, although labelled as a nursing model, is interdisciplinary in both its theoretical origins and application.

The Crisis Nursing Model is presented here as an example of a conceptual model for nursing practice upon which a community assessment might be based.

A summary of the four essential components of a model in the context of the crisis nursing model appears in Table 12.1. Stages of the crisis are outlined in Figure 12.1. A complete discussion of the crisis model is beyond the scope of this book and is unnecessary to the present discussion. For those interested in a description of the model and its evolution, see listing 21 in the Reference at the end of this chapter.

Table 12.1. Essential Components of a Nursing Model: Crisis

INDIVIDUAL (PERSON)*
  Physiological
  Psychological
  Social being
  Open system within environment
  Holistic
  Dynamic
  Active role
  Exists on orderly, consistent developmental continuum
  Existence: interrelated balance of external and internal relationships
  Participant: uses problem solving and decision making
ENVIRONMENTAL
  Internal and external forces
  Alters and is altered by individual
HEALTH
  Exists in relation to illness and environment
  Illness: prolonged state of disequilibrium or maladaptation
  Individual's perceptions affect definition of health
  Maintenance of equilibrium and successful coping are indices of
    health
  Wellness-illness-wellness model
NURSING
  Process based on sciences and humanities
  Augments coping behaviors
  Mobilizes resources
  Intervenes to prevent crisis, restore wellness
  Intervenes in crisis to restore maximum possible level of wellness
    post-crisis
  Process interactional
  Manipulates external or internal environment to help achieve or
    maintain higher level of wellness, prevent crisis
  Independent and interdependent functions

---

*Could be an entire community.

Figure 12.1. Stages of Crisis Theory*

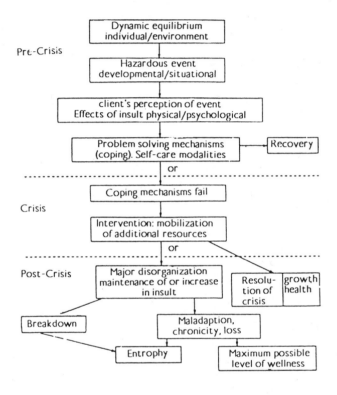

*Adapted from University of Connecticut School of Nursing, Storrs, Connecticut

In basing a community assessment on the Crisis Nursing Model, we must assess the stage of crisis represented by the community. Some communities will be in pre-crisis at the time of the assessment. Assessment may also occur in a crisis situation such as the planned closing of a hospital or an influx of new immigrants or refugees. Or it may occur post-crisis, e.g., in the aftermath of a crisis such as an earthquake, the closing of a local or public hospital or nursing home, or the closing of a factory or other place of employment through which workers have received health benefits. Such post-crises assessments resulted in the establishment of community health centers for primary care after the urban riots of the 1960s and 1992, and are occurring now in the aftermath of the failure of health care reform, a rush to managed care organizations and integrated care systems, and markedly decreased lengths of hospital stays, especially for dependent persons such as young children and older adults.

At times, there may be an overlap of community assessments conducted by public health (community health) or visiting nurses and other advanced practice nurses. Primary care assessments focus on the primary health care needs of individuals, families, and communities whereas public health field studies are broader in scope, encompassing primary, secondary, and tertiary needs of communities as a whole as well as of those who comprise those communities. Clinical nurse specialists may focus their practice on patients needing secondary and/or tertiary intervention (crisis or post-crisis). Nurse-midwives and nurse anesthetists focus on special populations. Any community assessment, therefore, requires that communication with health care providers within the community be studied to determine what assessments have been or are being done. In this way, duplication can be avoided.

Example: Pre-Crisis. The group to be assessed is the population of women over 60 in a New England semi-rural community. This community assessment was instituted by the local senior center's health advisor committee. The stage of crisis identified is pre-crisis.

1. Elicit the perceptions of those who can help gather data. These may include the potential target population for services, local health care providers, the director of the senior center, the dean of the school of nursing located in the community, town officials, and

social welfare persons.

　　2. Identify hazardous events, both developmental and situational, that are or may be present. Examples of such hazardous events appear in Table 12.2.

Table 12.2. Hazardous Events

DEVELOPMENTAL (MATURATIONAL)
　　Loss of reproductive integrity: menopause, processes of aging
　　Loss or threat to intimacy: loss of partner, diminished sexual
　　　　interest, declining sexual expression
　　Loss of relationships: empty nest, death of partner/mate, loss of
　　　　friends, retirement
　　Body image change: processes of aging
　　Responsibility for care of aging relative, grandchild, spouse, or
　　　　significant other
SITUATIONAL
　　Sexual assault
　　Accidents
　　Threat to or loss of: independence, mobility
　　Threat to or loss of body integrity: processes of aging; chronic
　　　　conditions in older adults; body image changes: mastectomy,
　　　　hysterectomy
　　Financial loss: retirement, death of primary wage earner, health
　　　　insurance

---

　　3. Factors that affect the potential for an optimal level of health must also be identified. These may also be called the resources available, both intrinsic and extrinsic. Table 12.3 lists some that might be identified.

　　4. Develop tools to collect data on the group targeted for the assessment as well as the resources in the community available to them and the women's own perceptions of their health care needs and their present problem-solving mechanisms.

　　Findings from the assessment may show that the services needed by the women might be included in one or more already existing agencies, or that new modes of health care delivery should be designed or new services created. An example might be a women's health center staffed by one or more women's health nurse practitioners located in a community hospital. Psychiatric and community health clinical specialists, gerontologic nurse practitioners, and other advanced practice nurses might be part of an intradisciplinary team.

Example: Crisis The community is a small rural setting. It is designated as one of the medically underserved areas of the country. The health care providers in the community include one family practice physician and several nurses with a variety of preparations,

Table 12.3. Factors that Affect Potential for Optimal Level of Wellness for the Community

INTRINSIC	EXTRINSIC
Genetics	Socioeconomic status
Nutrition	Resources
Ethnic origins	financial
Sex	social
	religious
	political
	cultural
	ethical
	health care
	Education
	Peers
	Family
	Significant others
	Environment
	home
	work
	social
	geographic

some of whom have not practiced in a number of years due to retirement or childbearing and child rearing. The family practice physician has just announced that he is leaving the area and no replacement has been found. The community has a high proportion of older adults who live alone on their farms or with younger family members, and many young families with small children. The primary occupations are fishing and farming. With so much surgery done on a day surgery basis and the early discharge policies of hospitals, community members are worried about care for those with serious illness, surgical sequelae, or new babies who are returned to the community. Coupled with this are expected cuts in health-care organizations and integrated care benefits for low-income families and the rush to managed care systems by many providers and agencies in the surrounding area. The nearest hospital is an hour away, as is the nearest nursing home, and both have recently been bought by a large for-profit health-care corporation. Most of the local physicians in that community have joined the corporation's managed care organization as providers. Hazardous events for the community appear in Table 12.4.

As an advanced practice nurse and member of the community, you suggest a community assessment might help to resolve the crisis

---

Table 12.4   Hazardous Events

DEVELOPMENTAL (MATURATIONAL)
    Aging of population
    Health care providers engaged in life development tasks:
        childbearing and rearing, retirement
    Young families with new babies and small children: single parents
    Older adults living alone or with younger family members
SITUATIONAL
    Loss of only physician
    No nearby hospital or nursing home
    Quick discharge policies of hospitals
    Decline in public monetary support for health care
    Usurping of local providers and/or agencies by outside for-profit
        corporation
    Move to managed care organizations and integrated care systems
    Many self-employed persons with no health insurance
    Welfare reform benefit limits

---

of the physician leaving. Community demographic data are readily available, as are data about health care resources in the surrounding area. This small community has the advantages of social support networks and other systems for caring for one another already in place (32). (See Table 12.5 for factors that support a resolution for the crisis.)

In the face of chaos in health care delivery, creative partnerships are possible between communities and health care providers within those communities (32). By examining the strengths and needs of this small rural community together, new partnerships

---

Table 12.5 Factors that Affect Potential for Optimal Level of Wellness

INTRINSIC
    Existence of community leaders
    Community dedication to helping one another and solving problems
        as a community
    Health care providers within the community
    Willingness of nurses and other health care providers to return to
        school to prepare for advanced practice roles
    Cadre of retired persons with skills and knowledge
    Community health center facility that belongs to the community
    Active community health council
    Effective social networks within the community
    Several trained and licensed home health aides available in the
        community
    Community ambulance service and trained EMTs
    Senior housing in the community
EXTRINSIC
    Active and innovative visiting nurse service with a hospice program
        for the area
    State medical school with a family practice program
    National Health Service Corps program for medically underserved
        areas
    Long-established relationships with hospital an hour away
    State university with satellite programs including advanced practice
        nurses

might emerge to tackle the problems. *Example: Post-Crisis.* The community to be assessed is a neighborhood in a city. The assessment area is ten blocks long on each side and bordered on one side by a large expressway and on another by railroad lines. The neighborhood is largely residential with a few small commercial establishments, mostly small grocers, package stores, bars, and cafes. Its inhabitants are mostly African-American or recent arrivals from Puerto Rico as well as long-time residents who are now elderly. Two local factories have recently closed, putting several hundred residents out of work there and in local businesses. Community leaders have identified the lack of available and acceptable health services as one of the critical problems facing the community.

Thus, the community has recently experienced a crisis, and is now in the post-crisis stage. Beginnings of resolution are identified by community leaders. As an advanced practice nurse, you are part of a group of health care providers called upon to do an assessment

---

Table 12.6 Hazardous Events

DEVELOPMENTAL (MATURATIONAL)
  Changing ethnic composition of population in neighborhood
  Deterioration of housing: tenements built 40 or 50 years ago
  Shift in prevalent age groups in population to adolescents and young
    adults and those over 60
  High birth rate, especially to teen population
  Single parent households: women heads of households
SITUATIONAL
  Unemployment rate high due to closing of auto assembly plant and
    jewelry factory
  Construction of 120 units of public housing two years ago without
    community consultation
  Completion of expressway cutting neighborhood off from downtown
  Retirement of only family practice doctor in neighborhood
  Political climate: threatened cuts in federal spending for health and
    welfare programs; welfare reform benefit limits

---

upon which to develop a plan for community-based health services. During the assessment process, it is important to elicit perceptions of both the crisis and the post-crisis state of the neighborhood from those affected and those who may be resources—community leaders, health care providers, and so on.

Hazardous events that may be identified for this community are listed in Table 12.6. Many of these have important implications for nurses as care providers. Some factors that will affect the potential for the people in the community and the community as a whole to obtain an optimal level of wellness are listed in Table 12.7.

In this particular neighborhood, several outcast groups are identified: new immigrants, adolescents, single parents, teen parents, and older and aging adults. Some of the hazardous events common

Table 12.7 Factors that Affect Potential for Optimal Level of Wellness

INTRINSIC

    Emergence of new community leaders; culturally diverse leadership

    Community dedication to rebuild grammar school, high school

    Three civic/fraternal groups with buildings

    Public hospital located within three miles of center of neighborhood

    Public transportation

    Community rooms in public housing projects

    Active visiting nurse and public health nursing services in city

    One school nurse with primary care preparation

    Three active churches in neighborhood

    Several vacant buildings in reasonable repair

    Active tenants' group in public housing units

EXTRINSIC

    Private foundation interested in funding primary care and new models of care for older adults

    Eligibility for National Health Service Corps provider(s)—designation as medically underserved neighborhood

    Interest in neighborhood health by professional schools in the city appropriate for nursing management. Examples include challenges of teen and single parenting, chronic diseases in elderly

    Plans for a major corporation to locate a division on periphery of neighborhood

to older adults, adolescents, and women are particularly appropriate to case management. Examples include challenges of teen and single parenting, chronic diseases, obesity, death of spouse/significant others and other losses, and diminishing abilities for activities of daily living. Nurses possess the background to understand the growth and development of all age groups and the skills to assist them.

Summary

The process of designing and implementing a community assessment with a community can be exciting and challenging. In addition to the obvious benefits of identifying underserved, alienated, and unserved individuals, families, and groups, caseloads may be increased, those not receiving any health care can be identified, populations of patients who have similar problems can be classified, and quality and quantity of care services can be increased. New models of care can be developed to meet changing needs such as movement of acute care from hospitals to the community.

An understanding of the complexity of events that impact on the health of a community and its potential for an optimal level of wellness can be gained through a more global perspective; the articulation between individuals who are concerned about the health of a community may begin with such an assessment; and the diverse views divulged may generate new ideas for resources to be tapped.

Advanced practice nurses have an opportunity to define the kind of practice they can be accountable for. A new image of nurses as professional health care providers can emerge. One way to further this process is to initiate community assessments in order to identify those for whom we are best prepared to provide health, illness, and wellness care.

REFERENCES

1. Waugaman, W.R. & Foster, S.D. (1995). CRNAs: An enviable legacy of patient service. *Advanced Practice Nursing Quarterly 1(1):21-28.*
2. Hawkins, J.W., Hayes, E.R. & Corliss, C. (1994). School nursing in America 1902-1994: A return to public health nursing. *Public Health Nursing*

11(6):392-401.
3. Taylor, D. (1998). Crystal ball gazing: Back to the future. *Advanced Practice Nursing Quarterly 3(4):44-51.*
4. Wald, L. (1915). *The House on Henry Street.* New York: Holt, Rinehart & Winston.
5. Dock, L.L. & Stewart, I.M. (1938). *A Short History of Nursing.* 4th ed. New York: G.P. Putnam's Sons. p. 33.
6. Breckinridge, M. (1952). *Wide Neighborhoods.* New York: Harper & Brothers.
7. Fuller, L. (1980). *Public Health Nursing in Chicago in the 20s, Reminiscences of a Visiting Nurse.* Unpublished material.
8. A statement on nurses in primary health care. *Primary Care by Nurses: Sphere of Responsibility and Accountability.* (1977). Kansas City, MO: American Academy of Nursing. p. 3.
9. Milio, N. (1975). *The Care of Health in Communities: Access for Outcasts.* New York: Macmillan, p. 57.
10. Bigbee, J.L. (1992). Frontier areas: Opportunities for NPs' primary care services. *The Nurse Practitioner 17(9):47-48; 50; 53-54; 57.*4
11. Nelson-Conley, C.L. (1990). Role development of the clinical nurse specialist within the Indian Health Service. *Clinical Nurse Specialist 4(3):142-146.*
12. Lamb, G.S. (1994). New delivery systems: The call to community. Unpublished speech delivered to the American Academy of Nursing Meeting, October 20-24, Phoenix, Arizona.
13. Ruybal, S.E., Baumens, E. & Fasla, M.J. (1975). Community assessment, an epidemiological approach. *Nursing Outlook 23:365-368.*
14. Smith,M.C., Barton, J.A. (1992). Technologic enrichment of a community needs assessment. *Nursing Outlook 40(1):33-37.*
15. Cordes, S.M. (1978). Assessing health care needs: Elements and processes. *Family and Community Health 1:1-16.*
16. *Rural Health Clinic Services.* (1979). Washington, DC: Department of Health, Education, and Welfare.
17. Hanchett, E. (1979). *Community Health Assessment.* New York: John Wiley & Sons.
18. An interview with Loretta Ford. (1975). *The Nurse Practitioner 1:9-12.*
19. Lytle, N.A., (1977). Jurisdiction of nursing: Areas of control and accountability in delivery of primary health care services. In: *Primary Care by Nurses: Sphere of Responsibility and Accountability.* Kansas City, MO: American Academy of Nursing, p. 21.
20. Mauksch, I. (Feb. 28, 1977). Unpublished speech presented at Boston College, Alpha Chi Chapter, Sigma Theta Tau.
21. Hawkins, J.W. (1983). Description, analysis, and evaluation of a developmental model. In: J.A. Thibodeau, *Nursing Models: Analysis and Evaluation.* Monterey, CA: Wadsworth.
22. Bozzo, J., Carlson, B. & Diers, D. (1998). Using hospital data systems to find

target populations: New tools for clinical nurse specialists. *Clinical Nurse Specialist 12:86-91.*

23. Doona, M.E., Sullivan, C. & Read, J.C. (1986). Psychiatric nursing origins and evolution at Butler Hospital, Providence, R.I.: Department of Nursing, Butler Hospital.

24. Doona, M.E. (1984). Nursing Revisited: The Worcester State Hospital and nursing. *The Massachusetts Nurse, January.*

25. Igoe, J. & Giordano, B. (1992). Expanding school health services to serve families in the 21st century. Washington, DC: American Nurses Publishing.

26. Ethridge, P.E. (1991). A nursing HMO: Carondelet St. Mary's experience. *Nursing Management 22(7):22-29.*

27. Hahn, M.S. (1995). The center for advanced practice. *Advance for Nurse Practitioners 33(4):45-47.*

28. American Nurses Association and the American Association of Occupational Health Nurses. (1993). *Innovation at the Work Site: Delivery of Nurse-managed Primary Health Care Services.* Washington, DC: American Nurses Publishing.

29. Barton, J.A., Smith, M.C., Brown, N.J. & Supples, J.M. (1993). Methodological issues in a team approach to community health needs assessment. *Nursing Outlook 41:253-261.*

30. Hjelm, J.S. (1995). The rural health care setting: Is there a need for a CNS? *Clinical Nurse Specialist 9:112-115.*

31. Stanley, J.M. (1993). NPs provide health care to homeless. *NPnews 1(2):1, 6.*

32. Bushy, A. (1995). Harnessing the chaos in health care reform with provider-community partnerships. *Journal of Nursing Care Quality 9(3)10-19.*

BIBLIOGRAPHY

Abraham, T. & Fallon, P.J. (1997). Caring for the community: Development of the advanced practice nurse role. *Clinical Nurse Specialist 11:224-230.*

Eng, E., Salmon, M.E. & Mullan, F. (1992). Community empowerment: The critical basis for primary health care. *Family and Community Health 15(1):1-12.*

Gauthier, M.A. & Matteson, P. (1995). The role of empowerment in neighborhood-based nursing education. *Journal of Nursing Education 34(8):390-395.*

Gauthier, M.A., Kelley, B., & Matteson, P. (1996). Introduction to the community through sensory information. In: *Expanding Boundaries: Serving and Learning.* Columbia, MD: The Corporation for National Service and Service America.

Hravnak, M. & Magdic, K. (1997). Marketing the acute care nurse practitioner. *Clinical Excellence for Nurse Practitioners 1:9-13.*

Kelley, B., Gauthier, M.A., Matteson, P. & Mahoney, M A. (1997). "Here comes the neighborhood." In: M.E. Tagliareni & B. Marckx (Eds.). *Teaching in the Community—Preparing Nurses for the 21st Century.* New York: National

League for Nursing.

Marion, L.N. (1996). *Nursing's Vision for Primary Health Care in the 21st Century.* *

Matteson, P. (Ed.) (1995). *Teaching Nursing in the Neighborhoods—The Northeastern University Model.* New York: Springer.

Matteson, P. (Ed.) (In press). *Teaching Nursing in the Neighborhoods: Innovative Responses.* New York: Springer.

Mezey, M.D. & McGivern, D.O. (1999). *Nurses, Nurse Practitioners.* 3rd ed. New York: Springer.

Rural/frontier Nursing. The Challenge to Grow. (1996) *

Stowe, P.A (1997). Starting a family practice clinic in a rural setting. *Clinical Excellence for Nurse Practitioners 1:105-109.*

Veeder, N.W. (1999). *Marketing Human Services.* New York: Springer.

---

*Available from American Nurses Publishing of the American Nurses Association: 800-637-0323.

ONLINE RESOURCES

Agency for Health Care Policy and Research (AHCPR):
www.ahcpr.gov
American Nurses Publishing: **www.nursingworld.org**
Centers for Disease Control and Prevention (CDC): **www.cdc.gov**
Food and Drug Administration (FDA): **www.fda.gov**
Management Sciences for Health (bridging the gap between public health problems and solutions): **www.msh.org**
Medicare: **www.medicare.gov**
Morbidity and Mortality Weekly Report: **www.cdc.gov/epo/mmwr.html**
National Center for Health Statistics: **www.cdc.gov/nchs**
National Library of Medicine (free access to Medline):
www.ncbi.nlm.nih.gov
US Bureau of the Census: **www.census.gov**
US Public Health Service: **phs.os.dhhs.gov/phs/phs/html**

Appendix A. Scope of Practice Statements, Standards and Guidelines and Role Definitions

Jordan, L.M. (1994). Qualifications and Capabilities of the Certified Registered Nurse Anesthetist. In S.D. Foster & L.M. Jordan (Eds.), *Professional Aspects of Nurse Anesthesia Practice.* (pp. 3-10). Philadelphia: F.A Davis.

Legal Aspects of Standards and Guidelines for Clinical Nursing Practice. (1998)*

NAPNAP White Paper. Educational Preparation and Role Parameters of Pediatric Nurse Practitioners. (1994) †

National Association of Pediatric Nurse Associates & Practitioners. Position Statement on Entry into Practice. (1992) †

National Alliance of Nurse Practitioners. Position Paper on Acute Care Nurse Practitioners (1995).††

National Alliance of Nurse Practitioners. Position Paper on Certification of Nurse Practitioners (no date). ††

Neonatal Nursing: Orientation and Development for Registered and Advanced Practice Nurses in Basic and Intensive Care Settings. In collaboration with the National Association of Neonatal Nurses. (1997).**

Nursing's Social Policy Statement (1995)*

Position Statement on Nurse Practitioner Prescriptive Privileges. (1996). American Academy of Nurse Practitioners.***

Scope of Cardiac Rehabilitation Nursing Practice. (1993).*

Scope of Practice for Nursing Informatics. (1994).*

Scope of Practice for Nurse Practitioners. (1992).***

Scope of Practice of the Pediatric Nurse Practitioner.†

Scope and Standards of Advanced Practice Registered Nursing. (1996).*

Scope and Standards of College Health Nursing Practice. (1997).*

Scope and Standards of Diabetes Nursing. In collaboration with the American Association of Diabetes Educators. (1998).*

Scope and Standards of Forensic Nursing Practice. In collaboration with the International Association of Forensic Nurses. (1997).*

Scope and Standards for Nurse Administrators. (1996).*

Scope and Standards of Nursing Practice in Correctional Facilities. (1995)*

Scope and Standards of Parish Nursing Practice. In collaboration with Health Ministries Association. (1998).*

Standards of Addictions Nursing Practice with Selected Diagnoses and Criteria. (1987).*

Standards of Clinical Nursing Practice, 2nd ed., (1998)*

Standards of Clinical Practice and Scope of Practice for the Acute Care Nurse Practitioner. In collaboration with The American Association of Critical-Care Nurses. (1995).*

(continued)

Appendix A (continued)

Standards of Community Health Nursing Practice. (1986).*
Standards and Guidelines for Professional Nursing Practice in the Care of Women and Newborns. 5th ed. (1998).**
Standards of Home Health Nursing Practice (1986)*
Standards of Nursing Informatics. (1995).*
Standards of Practice (1993)***
Standards for the Practice of Nurse-Midwifery.****
Standards and Scope of Gerontological Nursing Practice (1995)*
Statement of the Scope and Standards for the Nurse Who Specializes in Developmental Disabilities and/or Mental Retardation. In collaboration with the Nursing Division of the American Association on Mental Retardation. (1998).*
Statement on the Scope and Standards of Genetic Clinical Nursing Practice. In collaboration with the International Society of Nurses in Genetics. (1998).*
Statement on the Scope and Standards of Oncology Nursing Practice. (1996)*
Statement on the Scope and Standards of Otorhinolaryngology Clinical Nursing Practice. Developed by the Society of Otorhinolaryngology and Head-Neck Nurses and ANA. (1994).*
Statement on the Scope and Standards of Pediatric Clinical Nursing Practice. (1996).*
Statement on the Scope and Standards of Psychiatric-Mental Health Clinical Nursing Practice (1994)*
Statement on the Scope and Standards of Respiratory Nursing Practice. (1994).*
Telephone Nursing Practice: Administration and Practice Standards. American Academy of Ambulatory Care Nursing. (1997).
aaacn@mail.ajj.com   Online: www.iNurse.com/~AAACN
The women's Health Nurse Practitioner: Guidelines for Practice and Education. (1996). Developed in collaboration with the National Association of Nurse Practitioners in Reproductive Health.**

---

*   Available from American Nurses Publishing, 600 Maryland Ave. S.W., Suite 100 West, Washington, DC 20024-2751. **www.nursingworld.org**
**   Available from AWHONN, 2000 L Street N.W., Washington, DC 20036. **www.awhonn.org**
***   Available from the American Academy of Nurse Practitioners, Capital Station, LBJ Building, PO Box 12846,, Austin, TX 78711. **www/aanp.org**
**** Available from the American College of Nurse-Midwives, 818 Connecticut Ave. N.W., Suite 900, Washington, DC 20016. **info@acnm.org**
‡   Available from the Oncology Nursing Society, 501 Holiday Drive, Pittsburgh, PA 15220. **www.ons.org**
†   National Association of Pediatric Nurse Associates and Practitioners. 1101 Kings Highway North, Suite 206, Cherry Hill, NJ 08034-1912. **info@napnap.org**
††   NANP, 35 Pennsylvania Ave. S.E., Washington, DC 2003

Appendix B. Resources on Legal and Ethical Aspects, Credentialing, and Certification

LEGAL AND ETHICAL ASPECTS

State Boards of Nursing. National Council of State Boards of Nursing, 676 North St. Clair Street, Suite 550, Chicago, IL 60611-2921. Check state section in blue pages of telephone book.

Patient's Bill of Rights. Copies from American Hospital Association, 840 N.Lake Shore Dr., Chicago, 60611.

Code for Nurses with Interpretive Statements (1985). Pub. G-56.*

White, G. (Ed.). 1993. *Ethical Dilemmas in Contemporary Nursing Practice.* Washington, DC: American Nurses Publishing.*

CERTIFICATION AND CREDENTIALING

American Academy of Nurse Practitioners, Capitol Station, LBJ Building, PO Box 12846, Austin, TX 78711.
   Family Nurse Practitioner
   Adult Nurse Practitioner

American Nurses Credentialing Center, American Nurses Association, 600 Maryland Avenue SW, Suite 100 West, Washington, DC 20024-2571

Advanced Practice Clinical Areas:
   Acute Care Nurse Practitioner
   Adult Nurse Practitioner
   Adult Psychiatric and Mental Health Nursing Clinical Specialist
   Clinical Specialist in Child and Adolescent Psychiatric and Mental Health Nursing
   Clinical Specialist in Community Health Nursing
   Clinical Specialist in Gerontological Nursing
   Clinical Specialist in Medical Surgical Nursing
   Family Nurse Practitioner
   Gerontological Nurse Practitioner
   Pediatric Nurse Practitioner
   School Nurse Practitioner

Advanced Practice Nursing Administration Area:
   Nursing Administration, Advanced

---

*Order from: American Nurses Publishing, 600 Maryland Ave. S.W., Washington, DC 20024-2751. www.nursingworld. org

-- **(continued)**

Appendix B (continued)

The National Certification Corporation for the Obstetric, Gynecologic, and Neonatal Nursing Specialties, 645 N. Michigan Avenue, Suite 900, Chicago, IL 60611. Certification examinations for advanced practice roles:

Neonatal Nurse Practitioner—Registered Nurse Certified (RNC)
Women's Health Care Nurse Practitioner—RNC

American Association of Critical Care Nursing (CCRN) Certification Corporation, 101 Columbia, Aliso Viejo, CA 92656-1491.

American Board of Neuroscience Nursing Professional Examination Service, 224 N. Des Plaines, Suite 601, Chicago, IL 60661.

Neuroscience Nursing (CNRN)

Council on Certification of Nurse Anesthetists, 222 South Prospect Ave., Park Ridge, IL 60068-5790.

Certified Registered Nurse Anesthetist.

Board for American Occupational Health Nurses, 201 E. Ogden, Hinsdale, IL 60521.

Certified Occupational Health Nurse (Specialist) (COHN, COHN-S)

American College of Nurse-Midwives Certification Council, 8401 Corporate Dr., Suite 630, Landover, MD 20785.

Certified Nurse-Midwife (CNM)

International Society of Nurses in Genetics, 5775 Glenridge Drive, Building A, Suite 150, Atlanta, GA 30328.

Orthopaedic Nurses Certification Board, East Holly Ave., Box 56, Pitman, NJ 08071.

Orthopaedic Nurse Certified (ONC)

National Certification Board of Pediatric Nurse Practitioners and Nurses. 800 South Frederick Ave., Suite 104, Gaithersburg, MD 20877-4150.

Certified Pediatric Nurse (CPN): Nurse Practitioner (CPNP).

Oncology Nursing Certification Corporation, 501 Holiday Drive, Pittsburgh, PA 15220.

Advanced Certified Oncology Nurse (AOCN)
Oncology Certified Nurse (OCN)

Advanced Nursing Certification for Legal Nurse Consultants: Medical Legal Consulting Institute, PO Box 22778, Houston, TX 77227-2778.

National Certification Board for Diabetes Educators, 444 N. Michigan Ave., Suite 1240, Chicago, IL 60611.

Certified Diabetes Educator (CDE).

(continued)

Appendix B (continued)

Addictions Nursing—CARN Certification, National League for Nursing, 350 Hudson St., New York, NY 10014.
Certified Addictions Registered Nurse (CARN).
Board of Certification for Emergency Nursing, 216 Higgins Rd., Park Ridge, Il 60068-5736.
Certified Emergency Nurse (CEN)
Certified Forensic Registered Nurse (CFRN)
Certifying Board of Gastroenterology Nurses and Associates, 3525 Ellicott Mills Drive, Suite N, Ellicott City, MD 21043-4547.
Certified Gastroenterology Registered Nurse (CGRN).
HIV-AIDS Nursing Certification Board (HANCB), 11250 Roger Bacon Drive, Suite 8, Reston, VA 20190-5202. www.hancb.org
AIDS Certified Registered Nurse (ACRN)
Intravenous Nurses Certification Corporation, Two Brighton Street, Belmont, MA 02178.
Certified Registered Nurse Intravenous (CRNI)
Board of Nephrology Examiners, PO Box 15945-282, Lanexa, KS 66285.
Certified Nephrology Nurse (CNN)
Certified Percutaneous Dialysis Nurse (CPDN)
National Certification Board of Perioperative Nursing, 2170 S. Parker Rd., Suite 295, Denver, CO 80231-5710.
Certified Nurse Operating Room (CNOR)
Certified Registered Nurse First Assistant (CRNFA)
Plastic Surgical Nursing Certification Board, East Holly Ave., Box 56, Pitman, NJ 08071.
Certified Plastic Surgical Nurse (CPSN)
Rehabilitation Nursing Certification Board, 5700 Old Orchard Rd., 1st Floor, Skokie, IL. 60077-1057.
Certified Rehabilitation Registered Nurse (CRRN).
National Board for Certification of School Nurses, PO BOX 1300, Scarborough, ME. 04070-1300.
Certified School Nurse (CSN).
American Board of Urologic Allied Health Professionals, East Holly Ave., Box 56, Pitman, NJ 08071-0056.
Certified Urologic Registered Nurse (CURN).
American Academy of Wound Management, 1720 Kennedy Causeway, Suite 109, North Bay Village, FL 33141.
Certified Wound Specialist (CWS).

Appendix C. Evaluation Tool for Primary Care with Children*

	POOR	FAIR	GOOD	VERY GOOD
1. Synthesizes knowledge of life-span's physiological, sociological, psychological factors in primary care delivery				
a. Utilizes the theories of development when providing anticipatory guidance to parents.				
b. Is cognizant of the developmental, physiological, psychological, and sociological factors which necessitate specific planning and management strategies for children.				
2. Demonstrates continuing improvement with well-child assessments.				
a. Is able to conduct a history and physical exam with two children simultaneously.				
b. Is able to identify problems with growth and/or development.				
c. Administers DDST, immunizations and arranges for lab data with a sense of confidence.				
d. Relates to parent(s) and counsels appropriately re findings during the well-child exam.				
e. Arranges for follow-up appropriately with the help of the preceptor.				
3. Demonstrates continuing improvement in assessing and managing children with a specific problem (walk-ins).				

(continued)

Appendix C. Continued

	POOR	FAIR	GOOD	VERY GOOD

4. Integrates the responsibility
for the continuum of care for a
caseload of clients into the broader
role of primary care provider.
  a. Utilizes other health personnel
  when appropriate for commun-
  cation of care plan (i.e., social
  worker, school nurse, etc.).

5. Evaluates the total role of
primary care provider.
  a. By concentrating on well-child
  visits, demonstrates ability to contact with client at point of entry
  into the health care system and provide for follow-up
  and continuity of care from that
  point, assessing child within
  context of family/community.
  b. Integrates the role of primary
  care provider as teacher,
  counselor, and health promotor.

KEY:
  POOR: Inability to complete the stated objective.
  FAIR: Completes the objective, but requires much supervision
  GOOD: Completes the objective with minimal supervision or
       guidance.
  VERY GOOD: Completes the objective independently.

COMMENTS:

---

* Developed by Catherine Collins, RN, MS, and used with permission.

Appendix D. Advanced Practice in Women's Health Nursing II Clinical Evaluation Tool*

Please evaluate _____ (graduate student) by checking the columns marked "Exceeds," "Meets," "Below" or "N/A" as defined below.

Exceeds: Exceeds expectations for a student Women's Health Nurse Practitioner

Meets: Meets expectations for a student Women's Health Nurse Practitioner.

Below: Below expectations for a student Women's Health Nurse Practitioner

N/A: No opportunity to assess, no opportunity for student to demonstrate (please specify)

Clinical site _____

Clinical Preceptor _____

Dates of Experience _____

Performance Criteria	Exceeds	Meets	Below	N/A	Comments
Systematically and skillfully obtains complete health history and other information from available resources: • patient interview • available medical records & lab data • comprehensive physical examination • psychosocial, developmental and behavioral assessments					

* Developed by Amy Hochler, RNC, MS, and used with permission
Could be used for evaluation of a graduate WHNP in practice.

--- (continued)

Appendix D (continued)

Performance Criteria	Exceeds	Meets	Below	N/A	Comments
Utilizes comprehensive physical examinations, patient's history, signs and symptoms, as well as laboratory data to appropriately recognize normal and deviations from normal in body systems					
Effectively and appropriately orders and interprets diagnostic laboratory and procedural testing for women's care and treatment					
Makes appropriate and accurate clinical judgments and determines a prioritized plan of care in a timely fashion with each individual patient					
Performs routine diagnostic and therapeutic techniques accurately and appropriately within the scope of practice and standards of care for Women's Health NP's • physical and psychosocial assessment • speculum examination • pap smear/specimen collection • vaginal microscopy and interpretation • bimanual examination • post-op care • family planning counseling and management • hormone therapy • low risk prenatal care • postpartum care					
Utilizes knowledge of pharmacology to identify appropriate therapy based on findings from history, physical and lab data					
Effectively integrates health promotion, disease prevention, as well as normalcy of women's developmental and physical stages of lifespan into health care visits					

(continued)

Appendix D (continued)

Performance Criteria	Exceeds	Meets	Below	N/A	Comments
Effectively assists women by empowering them to make educated decisions about their own health care					
Demonstrates the ability to evaluate the appropriateness and effectiveness of treatment/ management with women at follow-up visits					
Identifies educational needs of women and utilizes skilled health teaching and counseling strategies with women of all cultural, ethnic, educational, developmental and financial backgrounds					
Able to recognize when health of woman is beyond the scope of professional practice and to refer or consult with other, more appropriate, health care provider(s)					
Demonstrates effective communication skills by providing a confidential, private, supportive, compassionate and respectful environment for women to receive care					
Effectively communicates and collaborates on or about practice concerns, knowledge and nursing literature with other providers					
Appropriately asks questions of other providers and uses information gleaned to provide women with more comprehensive care					
Documents findings and plan of care in appropriate format					

**Appendix E.   Sources for Information on Grants:
Nursing Organizations and Federal Agencies**

American Academy of Nurse Practitioners, PO Box 12846, Austin, TX
78711. **www.aanp.org**
American Association of Critical Care Nurses, 101 Columbia, Aliso Viejo,
CA 92656-1491
American Nurses Foundation, 1101 14th Street NW, Suite 200, Washington,
DC 20005. (Check your state nurses association also.)
National Association of Pediatric Nurse Associates and Practitioners, 1101 King
Highway N., Suite 206, Cherry Hill, NJ 08034   **info@napnap.org**
National Institutes of Health, National Institute for Nursing Research, USPHS,
Bethesda, MD.
National Organization of Nurse Practitioner Faculties, One Dupont Circle NW,
Suite 530, Washington, DC 20036. **nonpf@aacn.nche.edu**
Sigma Theta Tau International.   550 West North Street, Indianapolis, IN
46202. (Also check local chapter.)
Association for Women's Health, Obstetric, and Neonatal Nurses, AWHONN.
2000 L Street NW, Suite 740, Washington, DC, 20036. **www.awhonn.org**
Online.   NIH Guide to Grants and Contracts: World wide web
gopher://**gopher.nih.gov/11/res**
Oncology Nursing Society.   501 Holiday Drive, Pittsburgh, PA 15220-2749
www.ons.org
Department of Veterans Affairs, Washington, DC
American Psychiatric Nurses Association, 1200 19th St. N.W., Suite 300,
Washington, DC 20036

See also Appendix G

**Appendix F.   Guidelines for Prescription Writing Privileges for
Nurse Practitioners at a Community Based Multi-Service Agency
for Women**

Under Massachusetts State Law 105 CMR and agency policy, nurse
practitioners will issue written prescription and medication orders for
schedule III-VI controlled substance under the following guidelines:

  1. Nurse practitioners will meet all requirements for advanced
practice licensing set forth in Massachusetts regulations established by the
Board of Registration in Nursing.
---(continued)

Appendix F (continued)

2. Nurse practitioners' scope of practice will follow the rules and regulations for advanced practice under the Board of Registration in Nursing and the most recent guidelines for practice of the Association of Women's Health, Obstetric, and Neonatal Nurses (AWHONN).

3. Nurse practitioners will apply for and obtain a Massachusetts registration number and a federal DEA number.

4. Nurse practitioners will practice under a written set of protocols as agreed upon with the collaborating physician. New prescriptions and medication changes will be written according to the protocols for clinical practice or under direct consultation with the collaborating physician or his designee.

5. The supervising physician for the nurse practitioner named herein shall be Dr. _____ or his/her designee. Should the supervising physician be unavailable, the physician covering the practice will serve as consultant to the nurse practitioner until _____ returns.

6. Dr. _____ will review the NPs' prescribing practice, including all new prescriptions, via a review of the prescription log book every 90 days. This review will be documented in the prescription log book in writing.

7. Only schedule III-VI drugs will be included in the purview of the NPs writing prescriptions at this setting. NP prescribers will follow the regulations of the DEA and of the Commonwealth of Massachusetts with regard to the number of refills, duration of prescriptions and quantities of medications prescribed for all schedule III-V drugs.

8. All prescription pads for the nurse practitioners shall include the name of the agency, the agency's address, the nurse practitioner's name and registration number, and the name of the supervising physician.

9. A nurse practitioner may issue verbal prescriptions by clearly identifying herself, her professional designation, and her registration number, work address, telephone number and the name of the supervising physician to the pharmacist. A verbal prescription shall be followed with a written prescription mailed by the nurse practitioner to the pharmacist within not more than seven (7) days following the original prescription.

_____   _____   _____
Nurse Practitioner, signature   Printed Name   Date

_____   _____
Supervising Physician   Date

Appendix G. Nursing Organizations for Advanced Practice Nurses

American Academy of Nurse Practitioners. Capitol Station, LBJ Building, PO Box 12846, Austin, TX 78711. **www.aanp.org**

American Association of Nurse Anesthetists. 222 South Prospect, Park Ridge, IL 60068. **www.aana.com**

American College of Nurse-Midwives. 818 Connecticut Avenue NW, Suite 900, Washington, DC 20006. **info@acnm.org** website: **www.midwife.org**

American College of Nurse Practitioners. 503 Capitol Court NE, Suite 300, Washington, DC 20002. **ACNP@aol.com** website: **www.nurse.org.acnp**

Association of Advanced Practice Psychiatric Nursing, 5550 33rd Ave., N.W., Seattle, WA 98105.

Association of Nurses in AIDS Care. 11250 Roger Bacon Drive, Suite 8, Reston, VA 20190-5202. **www.anacnet.org.aids**

Association for Women's Health, Obstetric, and Neonatal Nurses. 2000 L Street NW, Suite 740, Washington DC 20036. **www.awhonn.org**

National Alliance of Nurse Practitioners. 325 Pennsylvania Avenue SE, Washington DC 20003

National Association of Clinical Nurse Specialists. 4700 West Lake Ave., Glenview, IL 60025-1485. **www.nacns.org** e-mail **info@nacns.org**

National Association of Neonatal Nurses. 1304 Southpoint Blvd., Suite 280, Petaluma, CA 94954-6861 **www.nann.org**

National Association of Nurse Practitioners in Women's Health. 503 Capitol Court NE, Suite 300, Washington DC 20002. **NPWHDC@aol.com**

National Association of Pediatric Nurse Associates and Practitioners. 1101 Kings Highway N, Suit 206, Cherry Hill, NJ 08034-1912. **info@napnap.org.**

National Association of School Nurses. PO Box 1300, Scarborough, ME 04070-1300. **NASN@mail.VRmedia.com**

National Conference of Gerontological Nurse Practitioners, PO Box 270101, Fort Collins, CO 80527-0101 **ncgnp@frii.com;www.ncgnp.org**

National Organization of Nurse Practitioner Faculties. 1522 K Street NW, Suite 702, Washington, DC 20005. **nonpf@nonpf.org**

Appendix H. Resume and Curriculum Vitae

SAMPLE RESUME
Name, Address
telephone, fax, e-mail

EDUCATION
♦ Boston College, MS Nursing, May 1999
♦ Framingham State College, BS Nursing, May 1997, Summa Cum Laude
♦ Community College of Rhode Island, AS Nursing, May 1984, Dean's List

CREDENTIALS
♦ MA License RN
♦ NCC Certification as a Women's Health Nurse Practitioner, 1999

Professional

Health Alliance Leominster Hospital   April 1996 — Present
Leominster, MA
♦ Staff/Charge Nurse in postpartum, nursery and labor and delivery

Boston College, School of Nursing   September 1998 — May 1999
Boston, MA
♦ Teaching Assistant - Community Health

Quinnsigamond Community College   February 1997 — December 1998
Worcester, MA
♦ Clinical Instructor - Maternal Child Health Nursing

Nurses' House Call   October 1988 — April 1996
Framingham/Worcester, MA
♦ Administrator, May 1994 - April 1996
   Total clinical financial and operational responsibility for large, full-service
   community health agency, including: budgeting, marketing, contracting,
   regulatory, quality improvement and management of multidisciplinary staff.
♦ Clinical Coordinator - Maternal Fetal Health, November 1993 - May 1994
   Developed and directed maternal fetal health nursing program for New
   England region.
♦ Clinical Nursing Supervisor, October 1988 - November 1993
   Case Manager for pediatric home care population, including: assessment,
   management of plan of care and supervision of direct care staff.

Milford Hospital   December 1987 — October 1998
Milford, MA
♦ Staff/Charge Nurse in postpartum, nursery and labor and delivery

(continued)

Appendix H (continued)

Woonsocket Hospital   June 1984 — April 1986
Woonsocket, RI
♦ Staff/Charge Nurse in pediatrics, postpartum and nursery

STUDENT NURSE PRACTITIONER CLINICALS

Southboro Medical Group   September 1998 — May 1999
Southboro, MA
♦ Women's Health Nurse Practitioner Student — Clinical Rotation

Jennifer Thulin, MD   September 1998 — May 1999
Natick, MA
Women's Health Nurse Practitioner Student — Clinical Rotation

HONORS/COMMUNITY/Membership
Sigma Theta Tau — International Honor Society of Nursing, Alpha Chi Chapter,
    Boston College
Framingham State College Nursing Honor Society — Steering Committee Co-
    Chairperson
Member of the National Association of Nurse Practitioners in Women's Health

PUBLICATIONS
Clancy, L. (in press). Would you like fries with that? Healthcare as a business.
    Clinical Excellence for Nurse Practitioners 3(6).

SAMPLE CURRICULUM VITAE
Name, Address
telephone, fax, e-mail

PROFESSIONAL EXPERIENCE

Massachusetts General Hospital, Boston, Massachusetts, 1986 — Present
    Clinical Nurse Specialist, Cardiac Access Unit, 10/98 - Present
        Clinical specialties include cardiac nursing and bioethics
    Per Diem Staff Nurse, Cardiac Access Unit, 10/94 - 10/98
    Per Diem Clinical Specialist, Department of Quality, Research and Staff
        Development, 1/94 - 10/94
    Cardiovascular ClinicalNurse Specialist, Surgical-Psychiatric Nursing Services,
        1986-1993
    Ethics Experience:
    Member, Optimum Care Committee, 1993 - Present; Member, Nursing Ethics
    Interest Group, 1987 - 1993; Chair, Nursing Ethics Interest Group, 1992 - 1993
                                                        (continued)

Appendix H (continued)

MGH Institute of Health Professions, Boston, Massachusetts, 19878 - Present
Clinical Instructor, Critical Care Specialty, Graduate Program in Nursing, 1992 -
1993; Adjunct Faculty, 1987 - Present
Boston College School of Nursing, Chestnut Hill, Massachusetts, 1990 - Present
Lecturer
Tewksbury Hospital, 1998 - 1999
Bioethics Consultant, Hospital Ethics Committee, 8/98-8/99
New England Memorial Hospital, Stoneham, Massachusetts, 1983 - 1992
Per Diem Critical Care Nurse, 1986, 1991 - 1992
Medical-Surgical/Critical Care Nurse Educator, 1983 - 1986
Atlantic Union College, Lancaster, Massachusetts, 1986
Clinical Instructor RN to BSN Program
University Hospital, Boston, Masschusetts, 1978 - 1986
Per Diem Staff Nurse, Coronary Care Unit, 1983 - 1986; Staff Nurse, Coronary
Care Unit, 1980 - 1983; Staff Nurse, Cardiothoracic Surgical Unit, 1978 - 1980

EDUCATION
PhD, Boston College School of Nursing, 1997
MS, Boston College School of Nursing, 1983
BSN, Salem State College, 1978

AWARDS AND FELLOWSHIPS
Boston College, University Fellowship, 9/93-5/96
National Institute of Nursing Research, Research Service Award, 9/95-10/96
Department of Veterans Affairs, Predoctoral Nursing Fellowship, 10/96-9/98
Harvard Medical School, Medical Ethics Fellowship, 9/97-6/98

RESEARCH
Doctoral Dissertation
Surrogate Experience: End of Life Treatment for Alzheimer Patients,
Phase 1: Completed 5/97
Surrogate Experience: End of Life Treatment for Alzheimer Patients,
Phase 2: 9/97-Present
Clinical Nurse Specialist for Improving Outcomes in Unpartnered MI Patients
(Principle Investigators, Drs. S.R. and D.C.) funded by National Institute of
Nursing Research, R15 NRO 4255, 1995-Present
Patterns of Morphine Utilization in Patients with Advanced Alzheimer's
(Collaborative effort with Dr. L.V., Dept. of Veteran's Affairs), 1/98-present.

PROFESSIONAL ACTIVITIES
American Association of Critical Care Nurses
American Heart Association:
Council, Cardiovascular Nursing 1990-Present

(continued)

Appendix H (continued)

Greater Boston Division Nursing Education Steering Committee 1987-1991
   Co-Chair, Steering Committee, 1990-1991
Task Force for Continuing Education in Cardiovascular Nursing 1984-1987
   Chairperson 1986-1987; CPR Instructor 1986-Present
American Nurses Association
Boston College Nurses Alumni Association
Kennedy Institute of Ethics
Sigma Theta Tau

PUBLICATIONS

List latest works first; underline your own name; primary author goes first; capitalize the first word of an article or book's title (and proper nouns); underline book and journal titles. Samples:

1. *Journal article with you (Ellen M. Doe) as first author, Stillwell Roe as second author, and Doody P. Coe as third author:*
   Doe, Ellen M., Roe, S. & Coe, D.P. (1998). Meeting the needs of unpartnered elders: A peer training program involving elders with myocardial infarction. Progress in Cardiovascular Nursing, 13, (4) 13-23.
2. *Journal article when you are not the first author:*
   Roe, Stillwell, Coe, D.P. & Doe, E.M. Advance proxy planning in patients who become incompetent. Federal Practitioner, 15 (5), 26, 29-30, 35-36.
3. *Your article in a book edited by someone else:*
   Doe, E.M. (1996). Informed consent: An important concept in patient education. In S. Roe and D.P. Coe (Eds.), Patient education: Issues, principles, practices (pp. 79-97). Philadelphia: Lippincott.

SELECTED PRESENTATIONS

Poster (most recent first)
Surrogate Experience: End of Life Treatment for Alzheimer Patients. Ellen M. Doe. Conference: Hospice Care for Persons with Advanced Dementia. Bedford VAMC, GRECC, Bedford, MA, April 1998.
The Impact of Ethics Rounds on the Moral Judgement of Staff Nurses. Stillwell Roe, Doody P. Coe, Ellen M. Doe et al. Conference: 7th Scientific Session, Eastern Nurses Research Society: Portland, ME, April, 1995.

Verbal (most recent first)
Nurses and Informed Consent. Ellen M. Doe. National Nurses' Week Presentation, Massachusetts General Hospital, Boston, MA, May 6, 1999.
Using Elderly Peer Advisors to Promote Health. Stillwell Roe, Doody P. Coe, Ellen M. Doe. Conference: Toward Research Based Practice, Dartmouth Hitchcock Medical Center, Nashua, NH, May, 1996.

Index